A Manual of

THE TREAT

FRACTURES

By

JOHN A. CALDWELL, M.D.

Professor of Clinical Surgery
College of Medicine
University of Cincinnati;
Director of the Fracture Service
Cincinnati General Hospital, Cincinnati

With 76 illustrations

1941

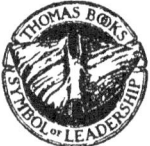

Springfield, Illinois

CHARLES C THOMAS

Baltimore, Maryland

THIS MANUAL *is dedicated to the House Officers
who have served on the Fracture Service of the
Cincinnati General Hospital in appreciation
of their help and interest.*

PREFACE

THIS manual of fractures has been prepared largely to meet the needs of medical students, house officers, and general practitioners. *The purpose has been to elucidate principles of procedure rather than to describe specific methods*—to try to rationalize what is considered good practice, and point out the errors in poor management. There has been a hopeful endeavor to help the seeker in understanding, in using his eyes, hands and reason instead of applying some specific gadget.

There has been no idea of supplying a substitute for the excellent complete treatises of Charles L. Scudder, Kellogg Speed, Wilson and Cochrane, Key and Conwell or Watson Jones. Free use and frequent reference has been made to all of these treatises in teaching, and in preparing this book, as also to Böhler's *Treatise on Fractures,* and to *The Management of Fractures and Dislocations* at The Massachusetts General Hospital by Philip Wilson.

The writer wishes to express grateful appreciation for cooperation, assistance, and encouragement to colleagues on the Staff of the Cincinnati General Hospital. His association with the successive house officers on the fracture service has been for some years his most pleasant and inspiring interest.

Miss Mary Maciel of the Department of Medical Art has been most painstaking and interested in preparing the illustrations.

JOHN A. CALDWELL

September 1941
Cincinnati, Ohio

CONTENTS

Chapter I

Varieties of fractures. Symptoms of a fracture. Repair of a simple fracture. Factors which modify union of fractures. Methods of treatment of fractures. . . . .

Chapter II

Anesthesia in fracture treatment. Comparison of inhalation, local, intravenous, and spinal anesthetics. Use of x-ray in examination of fractures. Methods of splinting fractures. Requirements for an adequate splint. Precautions to be observed in splinting. Comparison of splint materials. Restoration of function after removal of splints. . . . . .

Chapter III

Compound or open fractures. Types of infection to be expected and their prophylactic treatment. Treatment of compound fracture wounds. Expectant and radical. Dakin's treatment, Orr's treatment. Chemotherapy in bone infections. Gas bacillus infection. Chronic osteomyelitis.

Chapter IV

Fractures of bones of the face. Difference in healing of flat bones. Problems, deformity, obstruction of air passage and mal-occlusion of teeth. Fracture of ribs. Complications and treatment. Fracture of the sternum.

Chapter V

Fracture of clavicle—shaft and acromial end. Dislocation of sternal and acromial ends. Dressings. Fractures of scapula. Fractures about shoulder joint. Method of examination. Treatment of fractures of upper end of humerus. Dislocations of head of humerus—varieties—reduction and treatment. Fractures of shaft of humerus. . . . .

Chapter VI

Fractures of lower end of humerus. Other fractures about elbow joint. Principles of treatment of injuries about elbow joint. Fractures and dis-

Chapter XIII

Chapter XIV

Chapter XV

Chapter XVI

A Manual of
THE TREATMENT OF
FRACTURES

Chapter I

VARIETIES. SYMPTOMS. HEALING AND GENERAL CONSIDERATIONS OF TREATMENT OF FRACTURES

CERTAIN expressions are used in the description of fractures, each depending for its description upon the nature of the producing injury, and the location and the shape of the fragments. The following descriptive adjectives are in common use:

Simple fracture: One in which the bone is broken but the skin is not punctured.

Compound fracture: One in which the bone protrudes through the skin. These two expressions are not self-explanatory and are being gradually replaced by the preferable terms *Closed* and *Open. Transverse* and *oblique* are self-explanatory terms, for they describe the direction of the break.

A *comminuted fracture* is one in which the bone is broken into many fragments.

A *green stick fracture* is a break resembling one in a green stick. The bone is not broken clear through, but is bent.

An *impacted* fracture is one in which the force is applied in the long axis of the bone and impacts the fragments together. It nearly always occurs in the cancellous bone near joints.

A *pathologic* fracture is one occurring in a bone whose structure is weakened by some disease process.

SYMPTOMS

When a bone is fractured, the fragments are separated or displaced to a greater or less degree, depending upon the kind and direction of the force responsible for the fracture. When the violence producing the break is severe, there may be great displacement of the broken ends, with laceration of the soft tissues and hemorrhage about the fragments. This hemorrhage, combined with traumatic vasomotor paresis, may produce considerable swelling about the break and extensive ecchymosis; on the other hand, cracks in the bone (subperiosteal fracture) are associated with slight swelling and little ecchymosis. On inspection of the part, the swelling will be noted and also the position of the injured limb (which will be one assumed to restrict motion as much as possible). Deformity due to displaced bony prominences, angulation of a long bone, or rotation of the distal end may be noted.

On palpation of the part, one is struck at once by the rigidity of the muscles bridging the break and the resistance to passive movements. Attempts to manipulate the part cause pain and may elicit *crepitus*—the grating sound and sensation caused by the fragments grinding together. Crepitus is associated with much pain and *deliberate efforts to elicit this sign should not be made.*

Point tenderness: Pain on pressure (gentle pressure, preferably) *with the finger tips at the point of fracture* is one of the most valuable signs of fracture. *Stimson's sign:* Pain at the site of fracture on pressure in the long axis of the bone. This is another valuable sign, especially when the fracture is deep seated and cannot be directly palpated. Abnormal mobility or false motion is always present and is positive evidence of fracture when a single long bone is broken or two parallel bones are fractured. It may not be discoverable when the break is near a joint or the fracture is impacted or is incomplete.

The pain associated with a fracture is *dull and aching when the parts are at rest* and is due to the contusion of the soft parts and distension of the skin by pressure. *On motion, a sharp, stabbing pain is felt at the point of fracture* and is caused by tension on or tearing of the periosteum, which is the only part of bone carrying sensitive nerves. Some nervous diseases, e.g., tabes dorsalis, are associated with periosteal analgesia and patients, suffering from such disease, break their bones without feeling any pain. In manipulation of an injured part in which a fracture is suspected, *the greatest gentleness should be practiced.* Sudden, rough or forceful manipulation is certain to cause further muscle spasm and consequent pain, and induce timidity which makes subsequent examination just so much more difficult.

When the nature of the injury is not evident at once and careful examination is necessary, both the injured part and the corresponding part on the opposite side should be completely exposed for comparison. This is particularly important in injuries about the hip or shoulder.

REPAIR OF A SIMPLE FRACTURE

When a complete fracture occurs, there is separation of the bony cortex, the marrow and periosteum, and the surrounding soft tissues are lacerated or stretched, the extent depending upon the degree of displacement of the bone fragments. Under normal conditions the bone heals and becomes as hard and as strong as it was before injury, and the restoration is similar in every way to the repair of a wound in soft tissue by formation of a scar, except that in a wound of bone the scar must become calcified.

The new tissue by which bone is repaired is called callus and the deposit and ossification of callus may be divided into these periods:

1. The formation of a fibrin network, deposit of round cells and permeation of the mass by capillaries.

2. Organization of the mass into fibrous provisional callus.

3. Calcification of provisional callus into permanent callus.

Repair may be said to begin with the clotting of the blood which escapes from the torn tissues and a network of fibrin forms in the accumulated hematoma. Following this, there takes place the formation of connective tissue with the permeation of the mass by capillaries. In wounds in soft tissue, the structure of the scar is determined by the fibroblast. In osseous tissue, the osteoblast is the special bone forming cell which lays down the architectural design of the new bone. Springing from endosteum periosteum and bone marrow, it reproduces its own kind. At the time when osteogenesis is well established, a firm swelling will be felt at the site of fracture. The ends will be cemented together in a mass of tissue so that they will not easily be displaced, but the bone will bend at the site of fracture.

X-ray *at this time* will show nothing but the fracture, since the soft uncalcified provisional callus offers no obstacle to the passage of the rays.

The next step is calcification of the provisional callus. This is a diffuse process throughout the mass, causing it to become gradually more firm and resistant to movement. X-ray at this time shows a faint shadow about the ends of the fragments roughly fusiform in shape, which gradually becomes more dense.

The osseous callus is always formed in excess of the final need. Its quantity and form is determined by the amount of reparative tissue necessary to restore contour, alignment and axis of the bone. In laying down the pattern of causes, the osteoblasts seem almost to be endowed with architectural and mechanical judgment as shown by the fact that callus will be formed *on the concave side of a curve,* where it is needed to brace the deviated axis of the bone and will be withheld on the convex side.

In green stick or subperiosteal fracture or complete fractures perfectly reduced, *the quantity of callus* will be small. In comminuted fractures

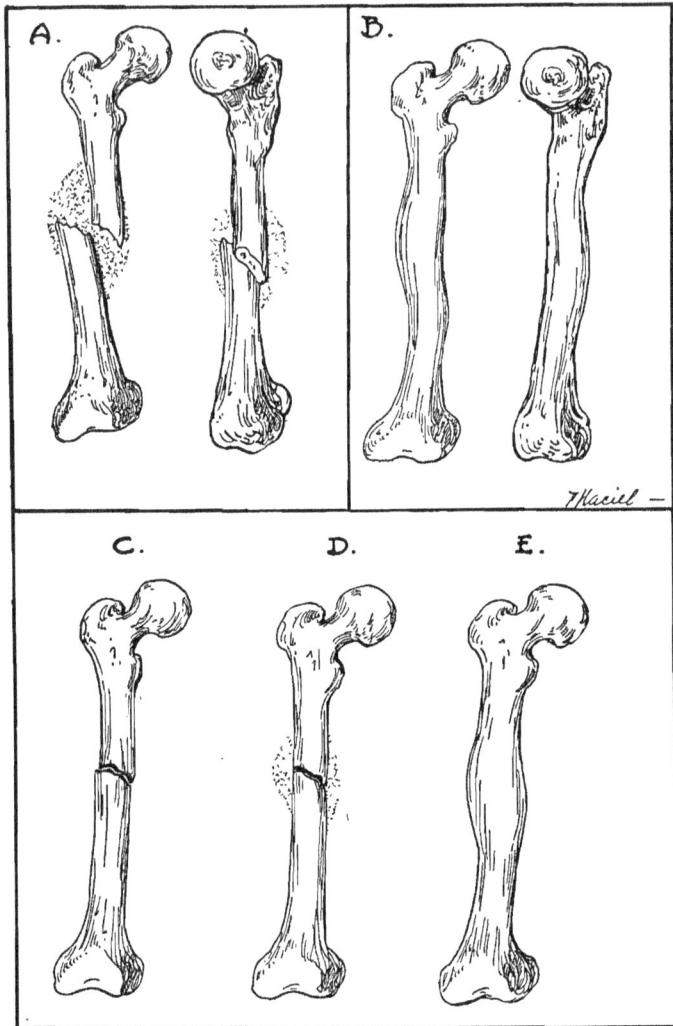

FIG. 1. Repair of a fracture. a) Fracture of a femur in a child aged 7, showing position of fragments and deposit of callus in 6 weeks. b) Same patient in 2½ years, showing absorption of excessive callus and rectification of the axis of the bone. c) Fracture of femur in adult aged 22. Practically perfect reduction. d) Same case in 8 weeks. e) Same case in 5 years. From x-ray tracings of author's cases.

or breaks imperfectly reduced, the entire shaft of bone will be imbedded in a mass whose diameter will be two or three times that of the bone. The appearance of a mass of callus about a fracture is often and very aptly compared to a wiped joint in lead pipe (Fig. 1).

The absorption of excessive callus (when the mass is very large, spoken of as exuberant callus) is brought about by a large polynuclear cell called the osteoclast. This absorptive process may continue for as long as two years until the new bone is reduced to the minimal size and shape necessary to restore strength and density equal to that of the rest of the bone. The x-ray picture at the completion of repair shows no evidence of the fracture but a more or less irregular swelling at the site of the fracture with the same or greater density than the rest of the bone.

The time required for complete ossification of callus (not absorption of excess and condensation of bone structure) varies from three weeks in a phalanx to ten weeks in a femur. The process proceeds much more rapidly during the period of life when bone growth is not complete, and during this period, astounding rectification of malalignment will take place and, frequently, shortening of a bone due to overlapping will be corrected by overgrowth of the bone to such an extent that the broken bone will become longer than its fellow on the opposite side. Other *factors which favor prompt repair* are good apposition, good blood supply and good general health. Comminution, poor apposition, impaired blood supply by injury to the nutrient artery, excessive associated soft tissue injury, and infection *delay repair.* Immobilization and constitutional conditions are factors in determining rapidity and firmness of union.

UNION OF FRACTURES

Certain fractures are known to carry an uncertain prognosis for union. These are fractures of the neck of the femur and the carpal scaphoid. Of the long bones, *failure of prompt union* is seen most frequently in the lower third of the tibia, next in the radius and then in the humerus. Failure or delay of union is uncommon in the scapula or ribs. The probable explanation of delay of union in some localities is impairment of the blood supply to the bone by the fracture. Interposition of soft tissue between fragments often delays or prevents union and separation of the fracture by too great traction is a common cause. Union is delayed somewhat when the fragments are not accurately brought in contact with each other, necessitating the deposit and ossification of a large mass of callus to unite them and, conversely, union is prompt when the ends of the bone are held in accurate apposition.

Local disease of bone is sometimes responsible for its failure to unite. The most common causes are osteomyelitis, tuberculosis, metastatic carcinoma, bone tumors, or bone cysts. Healing of bone is sometimes impaired by constitutional conditions. Of these, by far the most important are arteriosclerosis and rickets. Syphilis for many years was blamed frequently for tardy union, but since the Wassermann reaction has been applied almost universally, it has been found to have little affect, except insofar as it is a common cause for arteriosclerosis. Advanced tuberculosis may be an important factor in delay of bone healing. Diabetes and nephritis are often included as contributing factors, but these again when they have any influence probably cause it by the associated arterial disease.

Much of the impairment of bone healing is entirely without adequate explanation. Especially are the constitutional explanations quite unproven. The most baffling cases to explain are those of multiple fractures in different bones, some of which unite promptly while others prove quite stubborn. The most logical explanation in such cases is local interference with the blood supply.

TREATMENT—GENERAL CONSIDERATIONS

When a fracture is diagnosed, the first step in the care is to place the patient where appropriate treatment can be carried out. The best place is always a well equipped hospital where facilities for x-ray and anesthesia are easily available, but with some breaks, notably those of large bones with fragments freely movable, transporation and handling cause extreme pain and should only be done after temporary splinting to relieve motion. An anodyne is often indicated and, occasionally, local anesthesia is possible and is a most valuable way to relieve pain. In World War I a terse injunction became popular "splint 'em where they lie," and the value of this direction is constantly emphasized as time goes on.

When the patient is brought to the place of treatment, an x-ray should be taken to determine the exact location and the kind of fracture and shape of the fragments. This information is necessary in order to determine *the plan of treatment.* Most fractures can be treated by one of three plans:

1. Immediate reduction and fixation.
2. Traction and late fixation.
3. Open fixation.

1. *Immediate reduction and fixation:* By reduction is meant the replacement of the fragments so that the broken surfaces are in as complete apposition as possible. The common expression for this is "setting," and

it is popularly supposed that this should be done at once. Many conditions often prevent prompt reduction, notably great swelling of soft tissue, and it is rarely possible to reduce fractures which are not almost transverse. As a rule, anesthesia is necessary or desirable to effect reduction.

2. *Traction* is used when the obliquity of the break is so great that the fragments will not engage and the spasmodic contraction of the muscles bridging the break causes them to overlap. In these cases some form of continuous pull in the long axis of the bone is necessary, and this must be maintained until the muscle resistance is completely overcome and the fragments are fixed to some extent by provisional callus. Traction is made by means of an adhesive which fastens a strong fabric to the skin, or by skeletal traction. The common adhesives in use are zinc oxide adhesive plaster, mole skin plaster, Sinclair glue, Huesner's glue and celluloid varnish. Before an adhesive is applied, the limb should be shaved and cleansed with soap and water followed by alcohol. Painting the member with compound tincture of benzoin helps to hold the adhesive from slipping. The fabric is then applied evenly and smoothly and without wrinkles, *observing the precaution not to make pressure on a bony prominence.*

Skeletal traction is made by pins, wires or clamps fastened directly in the bone. Three methods are in common use:

1. Steinmann pin. A steel pin ⅛ to 3/16 inch in diameter (Fig. 2 a, b, c, d, e) is either driven or drilled through the bone and soft tissue and a horseshoe shaped handle is fastened to this and traction is made from it.

2. Ice tongs may be driven into the bone and traction made therefrom. (Fig. 2 h)

3. Kirschner wire may be drilled through the bone with a special drill, and drawn taut by means of a special clamp through which traction is made (Fig. 2 f, g).

COMPARISON OF TRACTION METHODS

Adhesive traction is easily applied anywhere and requires little special apparatus. It has the following objections: It is apt to slip and requires constant attention; many skins are irritated by adhesive traction which frequently causes great discomfort and often the treatment must be discontinued because of dermatitis and pressure sores.

The traction is made on the skin and not on the bone so that much

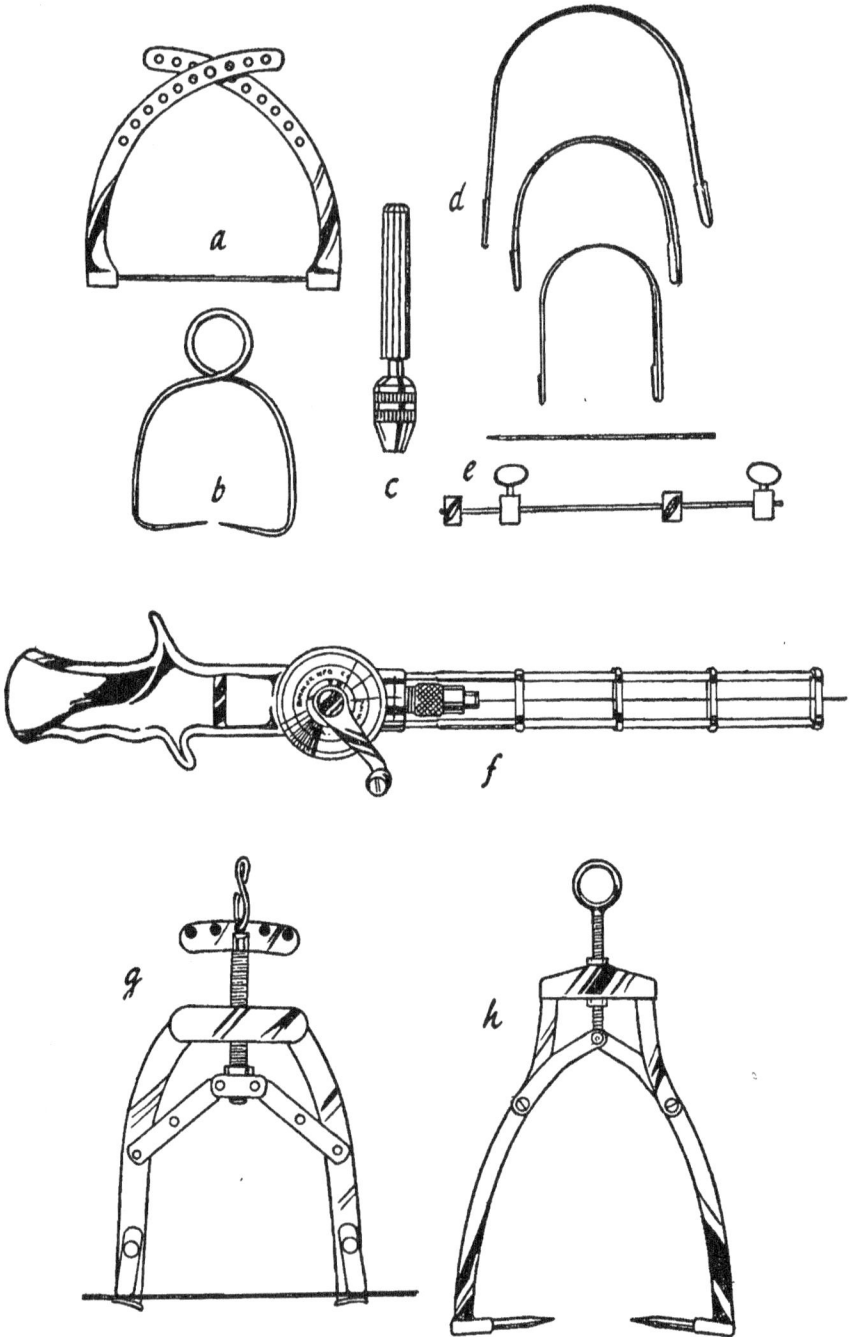

FIG. 2. a, b, c, d, e, f) Apparatus for skeletal traction. Drill for inserting Kirschner wire. g) Clamp for stretching Kirschner wire. h) One type of ice tongs. a, b, c, d, e. From the author's article: Treatment of fractures in the Cincinnati General Hospital. *Annals of Surgery*, 97:170, February 1933. Courtesy of Zimmer Manufacturing Co.

of the effect of the pull is lost through transmission of the force from the skin through soft tissues to bone.

The most comfortable and simplest form of traction is by means of a *Steinmann pin.* This may easily be inserted under local anesthesia since the periosteum is the only part of bone which has sensory nerves. It should always be drilled or spun through the bone, *never hammered through.*

Ice tongs and Kirschner wire are more complicated and expensive. Wire may cut through concellous bone in children, and the points of the ice tongs may penetrate deeper or slip and lacerate soft tissue. *Any form of skeletal traction should be applied with observance of rigid aseptic precautions.* The possibility of bone infection is always present.

REFERENCES

AIKEN, D. McCRAE: *Hugh Owen Thomas, His Principles and Practice.* London, Oxford University Press, 1935.

BÖHLER, LORENZ: *Treatment of Fractures.* Use of Skin Plaster. Wm. Wood & Co., 1936.

COMPERE, E. L. and ADAMS, C. O.: Studies of Longitudinal Growth of Bone. *J. Bone & Joint Surg.* 19, 4: 922, Oct. 1937.

MACEWEN, WM.: *Growth of Bone.* Glasgow, 1911.

MUNRO, J. K.: The History of Plaster of Paris in the Treatment of Fractures. *Brit. J. Surg.,* 23: 257, 266, Oct. 1935.

MURRAY, CLAY RAY: Healing of Fractures. *Arch. Surg.,* 29: 446-464, Sept. 1934.

MURRAY, C. R.: The Timing of the Fracture-Healing Process. *J. Bone & Joint Surg.,* 13, 3: 598-606, July 1941. Note: This article is followed by an extensive bibliography of bone repair.

SPEED, KELLOGG: Serum Calcium in Relation to the Healing of Fractures. *J. Bone & Joint Surg.,* 13: 58, Jan. 1931.

SPEED, KELLOGG: Skeletal Traction in the Treatment of Fractures. *Am. J. Surg. New Series,* 38, 3: 564, Dec. 1937.

TODD, F. W. and ILER, D. H.: Phenomena of the Early Stages of Bone Repair. *Ann. Surg.,* 86: 715, Nov. 1927.

WATSON, FREDERICK: *Hugh Owen Thomas, A Personal Study.* London, Oxford University Press, 1934.

WU, Y. K. and MILTNER, LEO J.: Stimulation of Longitudinal Growth of Bone. *J. Bone & Joint Surg.,* 19, 4: 909. 1937.

Chapter II

ANESTHESIA IN FRACTURE MANIPULATIONS. X-RAY IN FRACTURE TREATMENT. SPLINTS AND SPLINTING AND RESTORATIVE MEASURES AFTER SPLINTING

ANESTHESIA is usually necessary to reduce a fracture or dislocation. Its use may occasionally be dispensed with where the manipulation is obvious and simple and can be completed with a single quick movement. But it is often a mistake to dispense with anesthesia *when dealing with children* for the reason that the child may be immediately terrified and is non-cooperative when subsequent examinations are necessary.

Anesthesia is used not only for the purpose of relieving pain but to secure relaxation of muscle spasm in order that the bones may be moved upon each other and the ends brought into apposition.

Reduction of a fracture or dislocation does not, as a rule, require much time. Consequently, *an anesthetic which endures for some time is not desirable. Nitrous oxide* would be almost ideal, because of rapidity of induction and rapid dissipation, but patients anesthetized with nitrous oxide do not relax. *Ether* causes complete relaxation, but induction is slow and is followed by protracted nausea and discomfort. *Chloroform* is far more rapid, produces less discomfort and passes off more rapidly, but is *less safe* than ether. In the past few years two anesthetics—*Evipal* and *Pentothal Sodium*—have come into common use. These are rapidly acting soluble barbiturates which bring about unconsciousness with analgesia and complete relaxation very quickly. *They are particularly suitable for short anesthesia* and are comparatively free from danger. They would seem to be valuable aids for making possible painless manipulations of fractures and dislocation. They are administered intravenously.

For many years it has been known that a local anesthetic injected into the point of fracture would render the area painless, but the widespread adoption of the method was delayed and popular adoption was largely due to its advocacy by Lorenz Böhler. To be successful, the following technical features must be observed:

1. Two per cent novocaine or procaine should be used in quantities of 10 to 40 c.c.

2. The needle must be inserted into the hematoma surrounding the fracture. This is ascertained by drawing back the piston of the syringe after insertion of the needle and the appearance of pure blood in the solution will show that the needle is in the hematoma.

3. After injection, no manipulation should be attempted for at least ten minutes.

When two bones of a limb are broken both must be injected.

The advantages of local anesthesia are:

1. It does not render the patient unconscious.
2. Its effect persists for about two hours so that an unsuccessful reduction can be repeated.
3. The darkness and sparks present in the fluoroscopic room do not add any hazard to the anesthesia.

Local anesthesia is less effective in fractures several days old and is not so useful for reduction of dislocations.

Spinal anesthesia is often valuable for manipulation and splinting of fractures of the legs. It is not without immediate danger and occasional instances of cord or root damage are reported following its use.

THE USE OF X-RAY

X-ray examination of fractures is for the following purposes:

1. To determine if a fracture is present and to make a permanent record of its location and type.

2. To determine the degree of displacement, and the shape and the location of the fragments in order to plan the treatment.

3. After reduction and splinting, to discover if reduction is satisfactory and has been maintained.

4. During convalescence, films may be taken to ascertain if fragments are still in position and if callus is developing at the expected rate.

Obviously, many of these reasons overlap but one or more are always present.

An x-ray of a fracture or of a part containing a suspected fracture should always be made during some period of its treatment. Failure to do this is generally regarded as neglect or faulty judgment and is often evidence of malpractice unless x-ray facilities are unobtainable. *However, a patient should not be subjected to painful handling or shifting, un-splinted, just to get an x-ray for record only.* This is done too often where treatment must be carried out in a place other than the x-ray room. The proper arrangement is to have facilities for x-ray examination in the room where manipulation and splinting is to be carried out.

Fluoroscopic examination is often valuable in preliminary examination to observe manipulation and to check reductions after they are completed.

The fluoroscopic examination should never be considered sufficient in a doubtful case but should be checked by a film.

In general, the fluoroscopic examination is inferior to a film for the following reasons:

1. It does not make a permanent record.
2. It does not give the detail and definition of a good film.
3. There is definite hazard to the operator and patient from x-ray burn by too long exposure.
4. There is danger in prolonged anesthesia in a darkened room, and also the peril of igniting an inflammable anesthetic by a spark from the x-ray apparatus.

Too often the x-ray record of the fracture before and after reduction is considered sufficient and neglect to check a successful reduction several days later may prove costly, for an x-ray taken some weeks after the fixation dressing is applied may reveal that fragments have slipped. A most humiliating discovery is often made when a cast is removed several weeks after its application and there is disclosed recurrence of deformity at a time when fragments are too firmly fixed in their vicious position to be replaced except by an open operation. Such slipping of fragments is most apt to recur in fractures of the radius and ulna and the femur and tibia and fibula—*for no dressing can be applied that will prevent all movement of fragments.*

SPLINTING

A splint is a contrivance for immobilizing a part in which a fracture has taken place and so preventing displacement of the approximated fragments. It rarely can in itself prevent movements of the fragments but, by abolishing or inhibiting any muscle play in the adjacent muscles, it prevents them from displacing fragments.

Splints are of almost infinite variety and are made of many kinds of material.

An effective splint should accomplish these points:

1. Immobilize the joints both above and below the break in most

instances. This is necessary in order that all movements of the fragments —flexion, extension and rotation—will be prevented.

2. It should relieve pain.

3. It should not cause any pressure on bony prominences or unduly constrict the part to which applied.

4. In applying the splint *fingers and toes should be left exposed* in order that swelling or color changes due to constriction of blood supply may be observed and relieved.

5. It should move with the patient without permitting displacement of fragments.

Precautions to be Observed in Splinting

It is usual for some swelling to follow after a fracture has been reduced and a splint has been applied. If the splint has been too snugly bandaged, the ensuing swelling may cause great discomfort or even imperil the circulation of the part, consequently, this should be borne in mind and allowance be made in bandaging, and *the dressing should always be observed some hours after its application.*

An uncomfortable splint should always be carefully inspected to ascertain the reason for its discomfort. If the cause cannot be definitely found after examination, the splint should be removed and reapplied. *It is nearly always a serious mistake to administer an anodyne to relieve pain caused by a splint.* An anodyne may relieve the discomfort of the patient but the cause remains and may result in serious restriction of circulation which may even imperil the life of the limb, or pressure on a bony prominence may cause a local necrosis which will be slow in healing or make subsequent splinting difficult.

Splints when possible should be made of some material which is permeable to the Roentgen ray. This eliminates all metals except aluminum. Wood or fibre or pasteboard often make valuable temporary splints and they do not obstruct the penetration of x-rays. They are objectionable in that they cannot conform to the contour of the part.

By far the most useful splint material is plaster of Paris. This material is rubbed into the meshes of some fabric such as gauze, or crinolin, and this is then rolled into bandages. (Fig. 3) These bandages are immersed in water immediately before use and are quickly applied. This dressing hardens rapidly and forms a rigid splint which accurately conforms to the contour of the part.

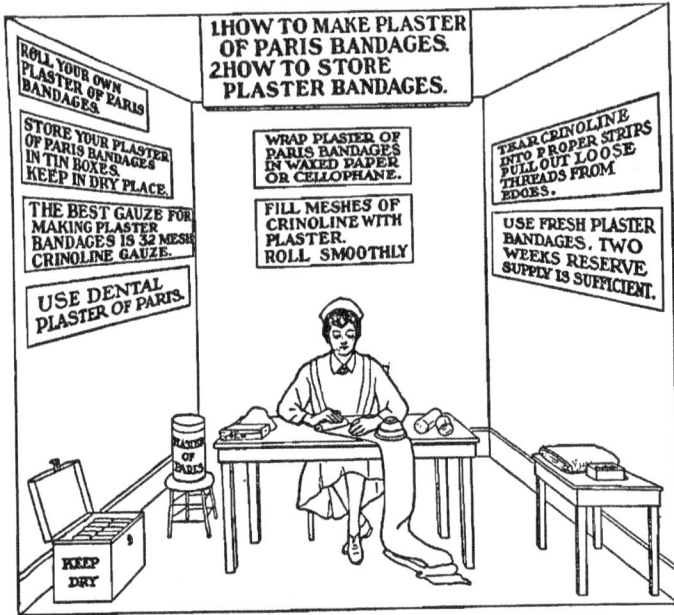

HOW TO MAKE PLASTER-OF-PARIS BANDAGES

Office and hospital home-made plaster-of-paris bandages are cheapest and best.

Buy 32 mesh crinoline gauze, tear it into 3 yard lengths, 2, 4 and 6 inches wide. Pull out three or more threads from each edge of the crinoline. Lay it on a table, fill meshes with plaster of paris of slow or average setting time. An earthenware bowl filled with plaster and inverted on the gauze strip is a convenient method of feeding plaster to the roller and steadying the gauze. Roll up the bandage by hand evenly and not too tightly.

At least one week's advance supply of plaster-of-paris bandages should be made. Wrap the plaster bandages in waxed paper or cellophane, folding the ends over and holding with a rubber band. Pack them in any dry receptacle as, for instance, a tin bread box, with a snugly fitting lid. Plaster bandages thus made and packed will keep fit for use for many weeks.

FIG. 3. How to make plaster-of-paris bandages. From *Primer on Fractures*. Cooperative Committee on Fractures. American Medical Association.

Two methods of using plaster are commonly employed:

1. Plaster splints. The plaster is laid out flat on a table or board, is applied to the part and bandaged in place.

2. The plaster bandage is wrapped about the part so as to encase it, forming a plaster cast or case.

With either method the plaster may be applied directly to the skin or the part may first be wrapped with padding (sheet wadding).

Skin plaster gives the most rigid immobilization, but certain precautions must be observed in applying it this way.

1. The skin must be free from abrasions, inflammation or defects.

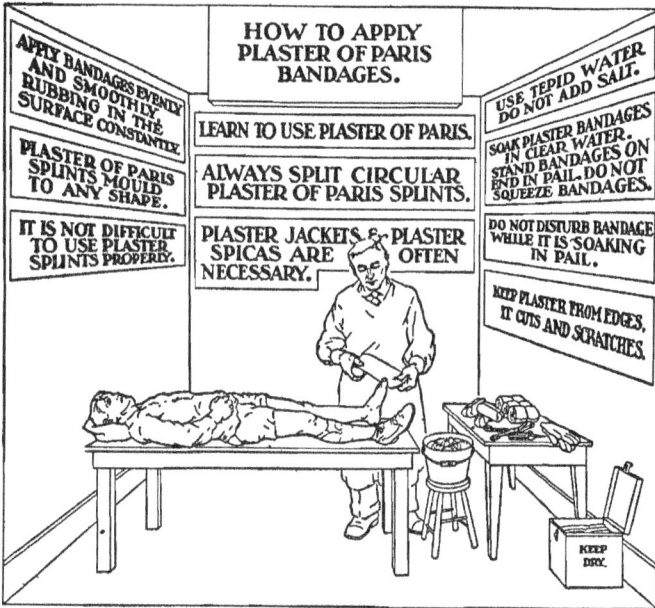

HOW TO APPLY PLASTER-OF-PARIS BANDAGES

Plaster-of-paris bandages can be made to fit a part of the body of any shape or size. Learn to use them without disturbing position of bone fragments. After removing the cover, place the plaster bandage end up in a pail of tepid water, deep enough to cover it. Do not handle or squeeze soaking bandages. When air bubbles cease to rise from the submerged plaster bandage, it is ready for use. Grasp it in two hands and compress gently to remove excess water but to retain plaster. Apply the plaster bandage by unrolling around the properly prepared and padded part, or make molded splints of suitable size on a table and bandage on immediately while soft. Apply the plaster bandage evenly without reversing, rubbing the layers smoothly on the surface. Reinforce weak points in circular splints with molded plaster bandages; not with any other material. Do not make the plaster dressing too thick; one-fourth inch is usually sufficient. Split circular plaster-of-paris splints to allow for swelling. Molded plaster splints can be faced with flannel just before applying to limb.

Fig. 4. How to apply plaster-of-paris bandages. From *Primer on Fractures*. Cooperative Committee on Fractures. American Medical Association.

2. Encircling bandages must be applied without tension so as not to deform the soft part and cause ridges or rough edges which are permanent when the plaster hardens. It is best, particularly for one who is not expert, to make the layers next the skin longitudinal or apply plaster splints and secure them by circular turns of the plaster bandage. *A "skin cast" should always be split its entire length as soon as it has partially hardened (usually in 20 to 30 minutes) in order that it may be spread or removed easily if it causes discomfort or much swelling follows.* It is extremely difficult to remove an unpadded cast without cutting the patient when the cast is tight and the plaster has hardened.

Edges of plaster dressing should be rubbed smooth or cut back or bound. Neglect of this may leave rough uncomfortable edges or may be followed by crumbling of the edges which may allow plaster crumbs to get under the cast or into the patient's bed.

RESTORATION OF FUNCTION AFTER SPLINTS HAVE BEEN REMOVED

After prolonged splinting, considerable muscular atrophy takes place as a result of disuse of the muscles; tendons grow adherent to their sheaths, and joint surfaces adhere to each other and to their synovial sheaths or coverings. As a consequence, when a splint is first removed, all movements of the part are limited in excursion, are painful, and are lacking in vigor. Much of this may be prevented by frequent changing of the splint and by judicious massage and passive motion.

After splints are removed, the above measures should be carried out with more vigor and the restoration of function may be hastened further by active movements; pain may be relieved and absorption of exudate may be hastened by frequent baking of joints.

When any change of dressings or of splints is made, the limb should be cleansed and rubbed with alcohol, and the part should be massaged gently. Any complaint of pain or pressure should be investigated, the splint being removed if necessary. *Under no circumstances should pain following the application of a splint be relieved with an anodyne.* Disregard of pain or treatment by blunting it with anodynes may permit a serious pressure sore to develop.

REFERENCES

DAVIS, LOYAL, HAVEN and GIVENS: Effects of Spinal Anesthetics on the Spinal Cord and its Membranes. *J. A. M. A.*, 97: 24; 1781, Dec. 12, 1931.

KEY and CONWELL: *Management of Fractures, Dislocations, and Sprains.* St. Louis, C. V. Mosby & Co.

SCUDDER, CHARLES L.: *Treatment of Fractures.* Philadelphia and London, W. B. Saunders, Eleventh Ed., 1939.

SPEED, KELLOGG: Philadelphia, Lea & Febiger, 1935. Chap. I.

WATSON-JONES: *Fractures and other Bone and Joint Injuries.* Baltimore, Williams and Wilkins, 1941.

WILSON, PHILIP D. and COCHRANE, WM. A.: *Fractures and Dislocations.* Philadelphia and London, J. B. Lippincott & Co.

Chapter III

COMPOUND FRACTURES AND THEIR TREATMENT. GAS BACILLUS INFECTION. CHRONIC OSTEOMYELITIS

OPEN or compound fractures are potentially serious deep infections and the problem of their treatment consists in management not only of the fracture but combating the ever present infection.

The bone in protruding always comes in contact with skin and clothing and often with the soil. There is always introduced into the wound not only the usual organisms of surgical infection but frequently the more dreaded and serious ones of tetanus or one of the gas-forming organisms (B. Welchi or B. Perfringens). These last are anaerobes and, when a grossly soiled protruding bone is replaced, there is danger of a deep-seated implantation of these organisms under anaerobic conditions which are favorable to their growth.

To combat tetanus, a prophylactic dose of anti-tetanic serum 1500 units should always be administered. This measure has completely proven its value in both civil and military practice and should never be omitted. Perfringens antitoxin should also be administered, though this is less certain as a preventive than the tetanus antitoxin. The two sera are now combined by most commercial manufacturers of serum so that a single prophylactic dose for both conditions may be given at once.

Before administering one of these sera, *always ascertain beforehand if the patient is serum sensitive.* This is particularly important in children, many of whom have had recent serum treatment or prophylactic administration of a serum for diphtheria or scarlet fever and are still sensitive to serum. When there is any doubt as to the patient's sensitivity, skin tests should be made before the serum is administered. *Neglect of this precaution may result in alarming or even fatal anaphylactic shock.*

The management of open fractures will be expectant or radical, depending on the amount of damage to the overlying soft tissues and the degree and kind of infection presumably present.

EXPECTANT TREATMENT

When the fracture has been compounded from within outward and there is only a slight puncture of the skin and there is no bone protruding.

The skin should be cleansed and shaved and asepticised while the wound is dammed off with gauze. The fracture should then be reduced and the wound should be closed and the fracture splinted as a simple fracture, except that in the splinting, provision should be made for inspection of the wound without disturbing the fracture.

RADICAL TREATMENT

Radical treatment should be carried out under general anesthesia and, when possible, in a hospital operating room.

It is to be employed when the fracture is compounded from without inward, when the bone is grossly soiled or dirt has got into the wound, or when there is great hemorrhage or severe damage to the soft parts.

The wound should be enlarged and all shreds and tags should be excised. Loose fragments of bone and badly damaged muscle should be taken out. This plan constitutes the operation known as "débridement" which came into extensive use during World War I. Following the operation the wound should be frequently and generously flushed with salt solution. Mechanical flushing and dilution of the infection is probably as important as antisepsis.

After these measures are completed, several plans may be followed:

1. *Closure.* This should only be done when the wound has been made very clean, when good approximation of the tissue can be accomplished without tension, and bleeding has been thoroughly controlled. When these conditions cannot be carried out, one of the following plans should be followed:

Dakin Treatment. The wound should be left open and several perforated Dakin tubes should be inserted in such a manner that all of the perforations will be buried and all recesses of the wound will be reached by the fluid. Dakin's solution should be instilled either by constant drip or by periodic instillation not less frequently than every two hours. When smears from the wound made on a microscopic slide show that the wound is free from bacteria, a delayed primary closure or a secondary closure may be made.

Dakin's solution causes an exceedingly stubborn dermatitis when it comes in contact with the skin for long, *consequently the skin should always be protected by spreading over it gauze impregnated with vaseline.*

2. *Orr Treatment.* The wound, after being gently but thoroughly cleaned, is left open and packed with vaseline gauze. Then a cast is applied, covering the wound and immobilizing the part.

The decision as to which of these plans to follow will depend largely on the experience and belief of the surgeon in charge and the facilities available.

Dakin treatment requires that appropriate apparatus and reliable Dakin solution be available, and that the nursing force have had some experience with such cases. *The Orr treatment* is simple, less irksome to the patient, but requires that the débridement and sterilization of the wound shall have been most thorough. An objection to this treatment is the extremely foul odor which always develops in the wound in about a week.

It often seems proper to reduce and fix an open fracture by some sort of internal fixation (plate, band, screws, or wire). It is rare that an infected wound will heal with a foreign body present. The temptation to employ one to hold an open fracture should be resisted unless the person responsible has had wide experience, seasoned judgment, and has at hand all facilities for carrying out his plan.

When in spite of thorough débridement and hemostasis (the most important deterrents of infection) this complication takes place, a condition supervenes which is full of possibilities for prolonged invalidism and peril to the future of the affected member. When bone once becomes infected, a portion of it is subject to coagulation necrosis and dies, and from then on it is a foreign body. Dead bone sloughs off very slowly and, while present, prevents both the union of the fracture and the healing of the soft tissues covering it. A fragment of dead bone is indicated by a sinus which refuses to heal and the opening to this sinus is evidenced on the surface by a crater of piled-up granulation tissue. When such a sinus is probed, the instrument comes in contact with hard bone, on which the exploring instrument grates as though it were in contact with stone. A roentgenogram will show a portion of the bone more dense than the adjacent bony structure and having a white appearance. This piece of dead sloughing bone is known as a sequestrum and after a time will become surrounded by a cloudy mass of new forming bone which develops about the dead fragment and may completely surround it. This growth is known as the involucrum. The entire sequence of events beginning with bone infection, followed by sequestrum formation and deposit of involucrum, constitutes the process called chronic osteomyelitis.

Gas Bacillus Infection

Gas bacillus infection results from deep implantation of one of the anaerobic organisms whose growth is associated with the formation of gas which distends the soft tissues. There are many of these, but that most frequently found is the Welch Bacillus.

These organisms grow best on devitalized tissue, consequently they are to be feared particularly when great soft tissue damage has been inflicted. When growth once starts the development of gas in the tissue causes pressure and so reduces circulation and causes progressive gangrene of the muscle.

Examination of the infected area shows it to be swollen with a bronze-like discoloration of the skin which is sharply demarcated. On pressure over the tissue there is felt the curious crepitant crackling of the infiltrating gas shifting under the compressing fingers. Gas may escape from the wound during examination when the characteristic sickening, sweet, putrid, odor will be noticed. X-ray examination of the part may show the gas infiltrating the tissues or accumulated in pockets in the muscle layers. Systemic symptoms are moderate fever, rapid pulse and prostration out of proportion to the fever and local condition.

The local treatment consists of wide radical opening to relieve tension and excision of all devitalized tissues. Probably the best local application is zinc peroxide. Kelly has reported effective inhibition of growth by frequent x-ray exposure. There is considerable evidence that chemotherapy, particularly the use of sulfanilamide and sulfathiazole are effective deterrents, and in all cases the polyvalent serum should be pushed. When in spite of treatment invasion continues, amputation is necessary to curb the progress.

Treatment of Chronic Osteomyelitis

The treatment of chronic osteomyelitis consists of immobilization of the part plus measures to ensure drainage, combat infection and favor the separation of the sequestrum.

Immobilization is best secured by a cast which must fix the joints above and below. A window may be cut in the covering plaster to permit drainage and inspection of the wound and the space between the cast and the limb must be carefully sealed with some water-proof material (vaseline gauze) in order that the cast shall not become foul from the secretions. When the sequestrum is well demarcated, it should be removed, and the wound left wide open and treated by *Dakin solu-*

tion, or packed with vaseline gauze and completely covered with the cast (*Orr treatment*). When the latter course is pursued, the patient's temperature should be the guide to the progress of infection. The foul odor which invariably becomes noticeable in a week or ten days is due to non-pathogenic saprophytic infection which, while disagreeable, is not incompatible with wound healing. Occasionally it may be advantageous to fix the bone by two or more Steinmann pins, inserted well away from the wound, and immobilization may be secured by clamping the pins to metal bars on either side of the leg.

Chronic osteomyelitis is always a slow process. Complete healing never occurs until all sequestra have been removed, or sloughed out, and subsequent recurrence of the condition by lighting up of latent infection is common. This may happen many years after the original infection has healed.

REFERENCES

BESLEY, F. A.: The Problems Involved in the Treatment of Compound Fractures. *Surg., Gynec. & Obst.,* 59: 354, 1934.

BULOWSKI, J.: The Orr Treatment of Osteomyelitis. *J. Bone & Joint Surg.,* 13: 538, 1931.

CARREL, A. and DEHELLY, G.: *The Treatment of Infected Wounds.* New York, Paul Hoeber, 1917.

DARRACH, WILLIAM: Compound Fractures. *Arch. Surg.,* 40, 5: 821-824, May 1940.

ELOESSOR, LEO: Treatment of Compound Fractures in War. *J. A. M. A.,* CXV, 1848. Nov. 30, 1940.

FOSTER, V. G.: Compound Fractures of Long Bones. *Surg., Gynec. & Obst.,* 56: 529, Feb. 15, 1933.

HERMANN, OTTO J.: Compound Fracture Therapy at the Boston City Hospital. *Arch. Surg.,* 40, 5: 853-866, May 1940.

KELLY, JAMES T., DOWELL, D. A., RUSSUM, CARL and COLIEN, F. E.: The Practical and Experimental Aspects of the Roentgen Treatment of Bacillus Welchii (Gas Gangrene) and Other Gas Forming Infections. *Am. J. Roentgenol.,* 31, Nov. 1938, 609-619.

KELLY, J. T. and DOWELL, D. A.: Present Status of the X-rays as an Aid to the Treatment of Gas Gangrene. *J. A. M. A.,* 107: 1114-1117, Oct. 3, 1936.

KENNEDY, ROBERT H.: Present Day Treatment of Compound Fractures. *Ann. Surg.,* 113: 942, June 1941.

KOCH, SUMNER L.: Immediate Treatment of Compound Injuries. *Illinois M. J.,* 67: 40, 1935.

LYLE, H. H. M.: Disinfection of War Wounds by the Carrell Method. *J. A. M. A.*, 68 Part 1: 107, Jan. 13, 1917.

McMASTER, PAUL E.: The Principles of Treatment of Compound Fractures. *Am. J. Surg. New Series*, 38, 3: 468, Dec. 1937.

ORR, H. WINNETT: *Osteomyelitis and Compound Fractures and Other Infected Wounds*. St. Louis, C. V. Mosby & Co., 1929.

ORR, H. WINNETT: Treatment of Compound Fractures. *Arch. Surg.*, 40, 5: 825-837, May 1940.

ORR, H. WINNETT: Wounds and Fractures. Springfield, Illinois, Charles C Thomas, 1941.

REYNOLDS, JOHN T., ZEISS, CHESTER R., and CUBBINS, WM. R.: Compound Fractures. *Arch. Surg.*, 40, 5: 844-852, May 1940.

SHERMAN, WM. O'NEILL: Treatment of Compound Fractures. *Arch. Surg.*, 40, 5: 838-843, May 1940.

SPEED, KELLOGG: *Open Fractures*. Fractures and Dislocations. Pp. 79-82. Philadelphia, 1935.

TRUETA, RASPALL JOSE: *Treatment of War Wounds and Fractures*. New York, Paul B. Hoeber, Inc., 1940.

WILLENSKY, ABRAHAM O.: The Value of Dakin's Solution in the Treatment of Acute and Chronic Osteomyelitis. *Ann. Surg.*, 75: 709, June 1922.

Chapter IV

FRACTURES OF BONES OF THE FACE.
MAXILLA. MANDIBLE. RIBS
AND STERNUM

FRACTURES of the bones of the face present a different problem from those of long bones in that they are not supporting structures but serve only as encasing protection to the soft parts beneath and as attachments for muscles. As a rule, fractures in such bones are not repaired by deposit of callus, *but are united by firm scar tissue.*

The principal undesirable sequelae to be feared are deformity, and obstruction of the air passages. Since fractures of these bones frequently break the continuity of the mucous membranes of the nasal cavity, the accessory sinuses, the mouth and the lachrimal duct, infection of the fracture and osteitis of the bones is a possibility.

These fractures are caused by severe direct trauma and are often associated with great laceration and contusion of the soft tissues. They frequently accompany fractures of the skull and may be a direct extension of such fractures.

The bones which may be involved are the palate, lachrimal, nasal, vomer, malar, and maxillary. It is rare that one alone of the bones is broken but combinations of several are more often encountered.

SYMPTOMS

Deformity may or may not be present, depending on the degree of displacement. It may be present, but concealed by the swelling of the soft tissues.

Blood may flow from the nose or mouth, or both. When the fracture communicates with an accessory sinus, emphysematous crackling may be present, owing to infiltration of the soft tissues with air.

FRACTURE OF THE LACHRIMAL BONES

The lachrimal bones may be broken in connection with the nasal bone, the maxilla or the ethmoid.

The principal problem in treatment is to remedy deformity and maintain patency of the lachrimal duct. The latter result is best brought about by frequent passage of sounds during the period of healing which is usually from three to four weeks.

FRACTURE OF THE MALAR BONE

This is a rare fracture alone and, when it occurs, is due to direct definite injury. When the bone is not depressed, no treatment is required. When it is depressed, it must be replaced or alteration of facial symmetry will result. Elevation is accomplished by a lever passed under the depressed fragment through an incision.

FRACTURE OF THE ZYGOMA

This is also a rare accident. When there is little displacement of fragments, no treatment is needed, but if fragments are much depressed, the scar and callus formed for repair may interfere with the temperomandibular joint. Such depressed fragments should be elevated by passing an aneurysm needle or strong wire beneath them and raising them into position.

FRACTURE OF THE MAXILLA AND MANDIBLE

These fractures nearly always communicate with the mouth and become infected, and an important feature of the treatment is the toilet of the mouth. Frequent rinsing of the mouth with an antiseptic wash is necessary, such as dilute hydrogen peroxide, potassium permanganate or Dakin solution.

Fractures of the maxilla are apt to cause deformity of the face, and when the fracture extends through the alveolar border, teeth to either side of the break may be loosened or so displaced that mal-occlusion of the teeth may result when the fracture unites.

Deformity should be corrected by moulding the fragments into place or elevating depressed fragments by means of a periosteal elevator. Loosened teeth should be pushed into place and held by wiring to adjacent teeth. When a section of the alveolar border is loosened it may be held in place by wiring the upper and lower jaws together.

Fracture of the mandible is caused by direct injury on the chin, or one side of the face, or by gunshot wounds.

SYMPTOMS

Mobility and crepitus may be elicited by grasping the lower jaw with both thumbs within the mouth and the fingers of both hands beneath the jaw. *Gentle motion* will cause pain, mobility and crepitus. If the patient is required to bite gently on a solid object (e.g., a wooden tongue blade turned edgeways), great pain is felt at the site of fracture. Since the principal disaster to be feared is mal-occlusion of the teeth, a dental surgeon is best qualified to manage such fractures.

A tooth in the line of fracture should be extracted. If allowed to remain, it will impede drainage and will almost certainly die and require removal later. The teeth on either side of the fracture should be wired together and the lower jaw should be wired to the upper. Occasionally an interdental splint should be fashioned and the jaws bandaged together.

The serious sequel to be feared is mal-occlusion of the teeth—consequently these cases are most understandingly treated by an experienced dental surgeon.

DISLOCATION OF THE MANDIBLE

Dislocation of the tempero-mandibular joint may be unilateral or bilateral. It may result from injury but usually results from contraction of the internal pterygoid muscles when the mouth is opened as in yawning. The mouth is held partially open and cannot be closed. The lower teeth extend beyond the upper. Swallowing and talking are interfered with. The mandibular condyle is felt as a distinct projection and a hollow is felt behind it.

REDUCTION OF THE MANDIBLE

The thumbs are wrapped and placed well back over the lower molar teeth and the mandible is grasped between the thumbs in the mouth and the fingers below the jaw. By pressing downward with the thumbs and upward with the fingers and pushing backward, the condyles are made to pass over the eminentia articularis into the articular fossa.

FRACTURE OF THE RIBS

Fracture of one or more ribs is a common minor accident as a result of falls or direct injury to the chest wall. Serious major injuries may follow collision, falls from a height, or cave-in accidents in which several ribs are broken and depressed.

SYMPTOMS

The most evident subjective complaint is respiratory distress. Any but the slightest respiratory excursion is apt to cause the broken ends to move upon each other, which pulls or pinches the periosteum or occasionally the pleura and this movement is associated with a sharp stabbing pain at the point of fracture, and the respiratory movement is suddenly terminated with a grunt. Coughing or sneezing causes a sharp stab at the site of fracture. Point tenderness is elicited by palpitation and may be emphasized by deep breathing.

Pressure on the sternum with the hand and counter pressure on the spine with the other hand, may cause sharp pain to be felt at the point of fracture (Stimson's sign).

X-ray for fracture of a rib is often negative and unsatisfactory, for the reason that many cracks are without displacement and the line of the ray is not at a suitable angle with the line of fracture to show the break.

COMPLICATIONS

Fractures of a single rib are usually uncomplicated, but occasionally a fragment punctures the chest cavity and emphysematous infiltration of the chest wall with air results. The subcutaneous tissues are distended with air, sometimes as far up as the eyes and down to the scrotum. Palpation of the distended skin causes the characteristic crackling in the tissue.

Major chest injuries may be associated with:

Emphysema of the chest wall.

Hemothorax.

Pneumothorax.

The last two are associated with laceration of the pleura or lung.

Later infection may convert a pneumothorax or hemothorax into an empyema.

TREATMENT

Since any respiratory difficulty is relieved somewhat by sitting up, patients with fractured ribs should be put in the Fowler position with as much elevation as they require to breathe comfortably. Morphine should be given to relieve pain and to slow respiration. A fractured rib cannot be splinted but the respiratory excursion of the chest can be restricted by a tight swathe of cloth or by strapping the side of the chest with adhesive plaster. For adhesive plaster strapping to be effective, the following conditions should be met (Fig. 5).

1. Starting from below, the entire side of the chest should be strapped.

2. The straps should each be pulled tight when the chest is emptied by expiration.

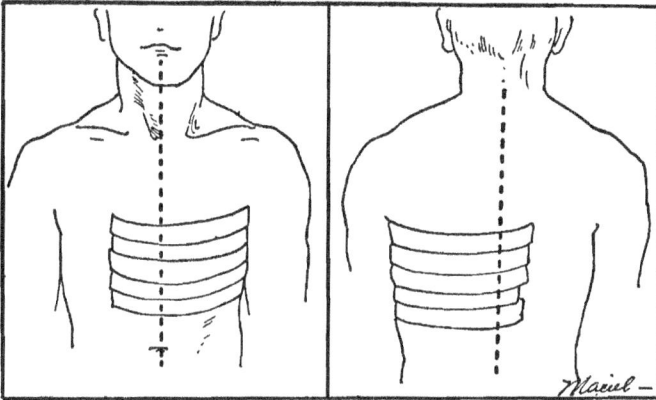

FIG. 5. Showing proper method of strapping chest for fracture of ribs. 1) Beginning from below each strap is applied and drawn tight at the end of exhalation. 2) The straps *must* extend beyond the midline front and back. 3) The entire side of the chest is strapped. The purpose is not to splint the fracture but to restrict respiratory excursion.

3. The adhesive straps should extend beyond the midline front and back.

TREATMENT OF COMPLICATIONS

Subcutaneous emphysema, though it causes a striking appearance, is not often serious and requires no treatment. Multiple punctures of the skin are quite ineffective to produce a general deflation, and make possible avenues for infection. The condition gradually subsides and leaves no sequelae.

Pneumothorax often causes sufficient embarrassment to respiration to require aspiration and this may be done as often as the air reaccumulates.

Hemothorax, if sufficient to seriously collapse the lung, should be followed by aspiration of the accumulated blood. It is best to postpone this for four or more days in order to permit the bleeding points to coagulate and some back pressure to accumulate and stop the bleeding. Early aspiration is more apt to require repetition than one which is delayed for some days.

FRACTURE OF THE STERNUM

Is usually caused by falls or crushes. The condition is often associated with fatal crushing of the chest or traumatic asphyxia.

In the less severe cases, there is localized pain aggravated by coughing, sneezing or attempts to extend the neck.

TREATMENT

Deformity is corrected by hyperextending the chest over a sand bag or edge of the table. Recurrence of the overlapping is prevented by adhesive strapping.

Rest in bed with the neck extended is usually necessary to prevent recurrence of deformity.

REFERENCES

Ivy, R. H. and Curtis, L.: Fractures of the Upper Jaw and Malar Bone. *Ann. Surg.*, 94: 337, Sept. 1931.

Moorehead, Fred B.: Fractures of the Jaws and their Management. *Am. J. Surg. New Series*, 38, 3: 474, Dec. 1937.

Shea, J. J.: Management of Fracture Involving the Paranasal Sinuses. *J. A. M. A.*, 96: 418, Feb. 7, 1931.

Stuck, Walter G.: Fractures of the Sternum and Thyroid Cartilage. *Am. J. Surg. New Series*, 38, 3: 560.

Chapter V

FRACTURES OF CLAVICLE, SCAPULA, AND HUMERUS ABOUT SHOULDER JOINT. DISLOCATIONS OF SHOULDER. FRACTURES OF SHAFT OF HUMERUS

T HE clavicle is one of the bones most frequently broken. The most common site of breakage is at the junction of the outer and middle thirds *where the diameter of the bone is smallest.* The cause is usually a fall upon the shoulder or the outstretched hand. *The fracture is apt to be oblique,* rather than transverse. Green-stick fracture is common in children.

Fractures of the shaft of the clavicle are difficult to reduce and then quite troublesome to maintain in position. This is owing to the impossibility of completely immobilizing the shoulder and the constant movements of respiration. Probably no fracture has had so many appliances and methods for its fixation described, which indicates that none has proved entirely satisfactory. While perfect reposition of fragments does not usually follow attempts at reduction, marked deformity, failure of union and impaired function are rare sequels.

SYMPTOMS

The affected shoulder droops and the inner fragment is pulled upward by the action of the sternomastoid muscle. Reduction is affected

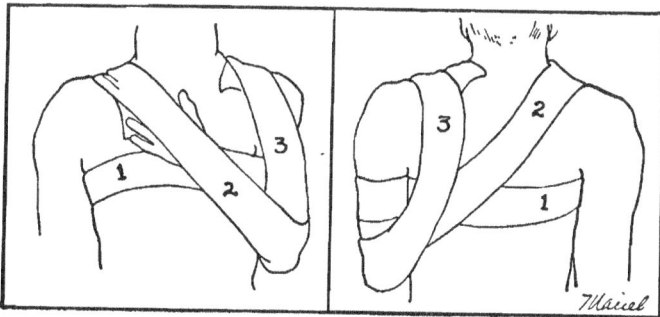

FIG. 6. Sayer's dressing for fracture of the clavicle. Excellent for reducing and holding marked displacement. It is very uncomfortable and rarely tolerated for long.

31

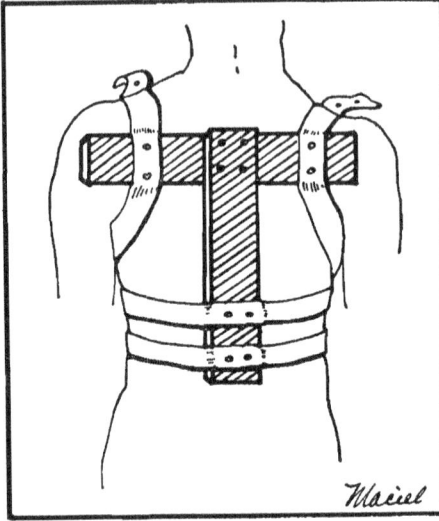

FIG. 7. Clavicle brace. Comfortable. Fairly effective and easily changed. Can be worn under clothing.

by drawing the shoulder upward and back, and all of the methods of fixation are based on maintaining this position. The common dressings are Valpeau, Sayers (Fig. 6), Clavicular cross (Fig. 7), Figure-of-eight (Fig. 8), Jockey strap (Fig. 9).

The best method is rest in bed and this yields the most satisfactory results, but can rarely be applied except when the fractured clavicle is associated with severe injuries. Any dressing should be worn for four weeks and the forearm carried in a sling for two weeks more.

Sterno-clavicular dislocation is usually upward and caused by violent depression of the shoulder. The head of the bone projects above and forward and is quite painful. Reduction is affected by placing the op-

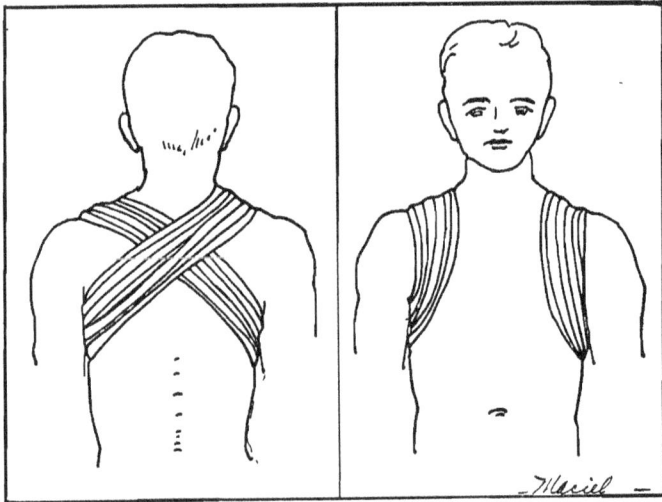

FIG. 8. Figure-of-eight bandages. Not very effective. Soon loosened and must be changed frequently.

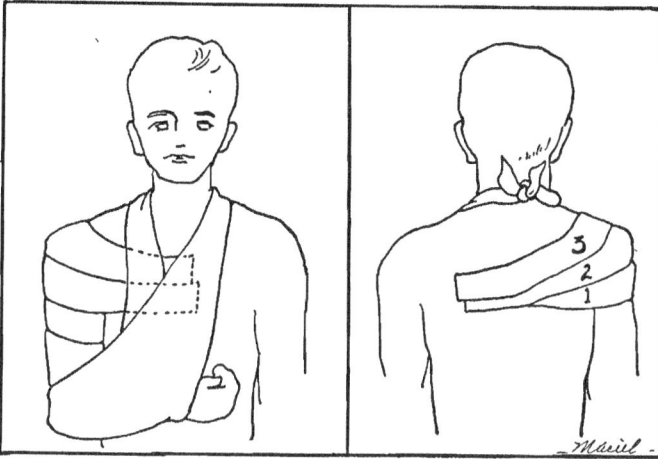

FIG. 9. Jockey strap dressing for fracture of the clavicle. Easily applied. Comfortable and effective. Can be worn under clothing.

erator's knee between the shoulder, his foot on the seat of the patient's chair. The shoulders are drawn back forcibly and the bone is manipulated into position. Reduction is as a rule easy but often difficult to maintain. Recumbency is frequently necessary to keep the head in position. Open operation, repair of the capsule, or some forms of anchorage of the head in position is often necessary.

Fracture of the acromial end of the clavicle within the acromio-clavicular ligament sometimes occurs and often without displacement. The diagnosis is made by point tenderness and x-ray.

No dressing is necessary in most instances, but a sling for the forearm to take the weight off the shoulder and restrict movement gives comfort.

Dislocation of the acromial end upward (Fig. 10) is an occasional accident.

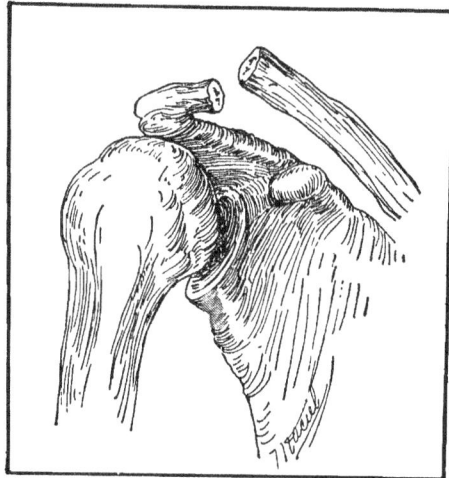

FIG. 10. Dislocation of the acromial end of the clavicle. Constant type of displacement easily reduced but difficult to maintain in position. Fixation by open operation often necessary.

The shoulder droops. There is an asymmetric prominence just medial to the acromion. This prominence may be obliterated by pressing downward but recurs as soon as pressure is removed. This dislocation is extremely difficult to maintain in reduction. The most successful dressing is the "trunk strap" (Fig. 11), but this must be watched carefully and adjusted frequently. Adhesive plaster directly on the skin is inadvisable, for the reason that open operation is frequently necessary and an adhesive plaster dermatitis may make operative measures impossible for some time.

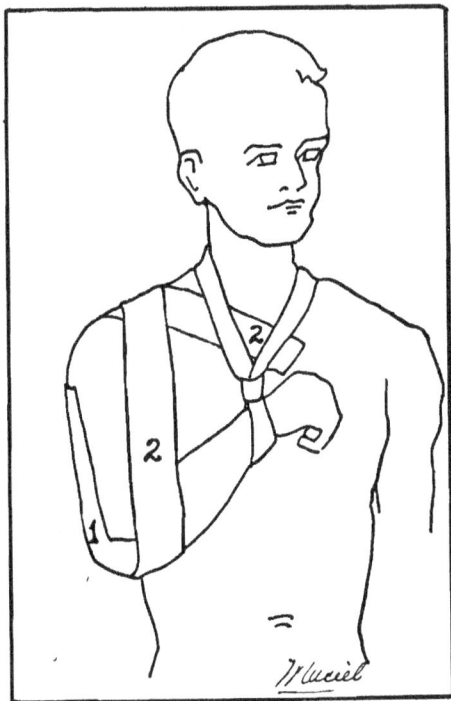

FIG. 11. Nichols and Smith's dressing for dislocation of acromial end of clavicle.

Open operation should be done in all cases where reduction cannot be maintained for failure of reduction is followed by considerable disability and discomfort. Simple wiring or anchorage with absorbable material is not sufficient in most instances. *Proper operation consists in* restoring the capsule of the acromic-clavicular joint and also the coraco-acromial ligament. One of the best operations for correcting this condition has been described by Sterling Bunnell.

FRACTURE OF THE SCAPULA

Since the scapula is freely movable and is suspended in muscles, fracture occurs only by direct violence and then the injury must be a severe one.

The following varieties have been seen, usually several are present at the same time:

1. Through glenoid fossa.
2. Body.

3. Angles.
4. Acromion.
5. Coracoid process.
6. Neck.

The prominent symptoms are swelling and pain on movement of the shoulder. Crepitus may be elicited but is frequently absent. A definite diagnosis is often impossible until good stereoscopic x-ray films have been taken.

Reduction is often impossible and an open fixation is rarely justified.

TREATMENT

Some method of immobilization of the shoulder joint is required. Occasionally recumbency in bed, with some form of traction on the humerus, will be necessary. Cracks without any or slight displacement may be treated easiest by fixing the arm to the side with a swathe. If the break requires prolonged immobilization, the arm should be abducted by a spica cast, an aeroplane splint, or Mittledorph triangle.

FRACTURE ABOUT THE SHOULDER JOINT

In addition to the fracture and dislocation of the acromial end of the clavicle and fractures of the scapula, the following types of injury may occur about the shoulder joint:

1. Contusion of the shoulder.
2. Fracture of the surgical neck of the humerus.
3. Separation of the upper epiphysis of the humerus.
4. Fracture of the anatomic neck of the humerus.
5. Dislocation of the head of the humerus.
6. Fractures of the greater tuberosity of the humerus.

METHOD OF EXAMINATION

Both shoulders should be symmetrically exposed and carefully compared for both front and rear. The particular points to note are:

1. Abnormal swelling.
2. Presence of abnormal prominence.
3. Absence of a normal prominence.
4. Deviation of the normal axis of the humerus.
5. Alteration of the direction of the axis of the humerus.

By palpation one should:

1. Check observations 1, 2 and 3 above.

2. Grasp the head of the humerus between the thumb in front and the fingers behind. Then gently rotate the head of the humerus by sweeping the flexed forearm to and fro across the chest.

Note: 1. If the head rotates with the shaft of the bone.

2. If crepitus is felt.

Stimson's Sign: Place one hand on the acromion and head of the humerus, the other on the elbow. Press the two hands together. A positive Stimson's sign is manifested by sharp pain at the site of fracture. Since the upper fragment is short and deeply buried in muscle, abnormal mobility and angulation may be difficult or impossible to elicit.

FRACTURE OF THE SURGICAL NECK OF THE HUMERUS (FIG. 12)

This is a frequent injury, *more common after middle life.*

A subperiosteal fracture is often seen in children. When displacement occurs, the common condition is for the upper end of the shaft to be pulled inward by the pectoralis major while the head is rotated outward and forward by the supra and infraspinatus and teres minor. When impacted in good position, a diagnosis may be impossible without x-ray. When fragments are displaced, the following conditions are present:

1. The shoulder is swollen but the head of the humerus is in the glinoid cavity.

2. The axis of the humerus may point inward.

3. The head of the bone does not rotate with the shaft, and attempts to determine this may elicit crepitus.

4. Stimson's sign is positive just below the head of the bone.

Reduction is attempted by traction and manipulation but is not attended by a high proportion of success for the reason that the head and neck are covered with such a deep pad of muscle that it is impossible to fix them sufficiently or to make counter traction.

Fracture of the anatomic neck of the humerus is a much less frequent injury than that of the surgical neck. It is most often seen in elderly patients. The position and displacement are similar, and what was said about reduction of the lower fracture applies to this one also. It is frequently impacted. Splinting and treatment will be considered with the other injuries about the shoulder joint.

Separation of the upper epiphysis of the humerus is similar in every way to fracture of the surgical neck. It is an occasional birth injury and may occur at any time from birth to the sixteenth year. What was said about fractures of the surgical neck concerning symptoms and reduction

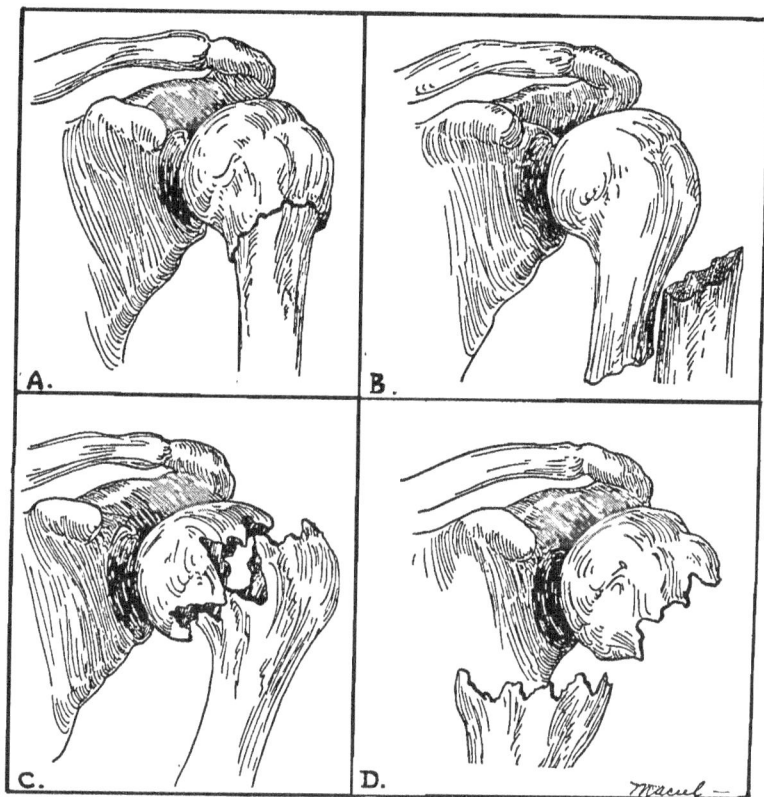

FIG. 12. Fractures of upper end of humerus. Showing commoner types and displacements.
a) Impacted surgical neck. b) Neck displaced toward axilla. c) Fracture of anatomical
neck without displacement rotated outward and upward. Shaft outside. d) Fracture of
anatomical neck with displacement.

FIG. 13. Separation of greater tuberosity. May result from direct injury or
avulsion. Often associated with anterior
dislocation.

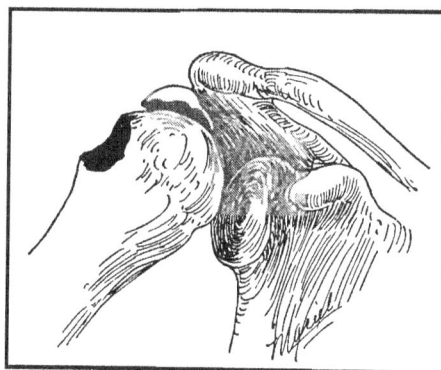

applies to this injury also. Treatment will be considered with other injuries about the shoulder joint.

Separation of the upper epiphysis is occasionally followed by impaired growth of the humerus which results in shortening of the injured arm. This sequel is more apt to follow when reduction has not been complete.

Fracture of the greater tuberosity (Fig. 13). This accident may follow direct violence from falls on the shoulder and may also result from avulsion of the prominence by contraction of the attached muscles.

SYMPTOMS

The shoulder is swollen and there is extreme tenderness on pressure over the tuberosity. Attempts to abduct or externally rotate the arms cause sharp pain over the tip of the shoulder. This injury cannot be positively diagnosed from a contusion or other fractures about the shoulder except by x-ray.

TREATMENT OF FRACTURES OF THE HUMERUS ABOUT THE SHOULDER JOINT

When the fracture is in the shaft and impacted or can be reduced, it may be splinted in one of two ways. The arm should be firmly bound

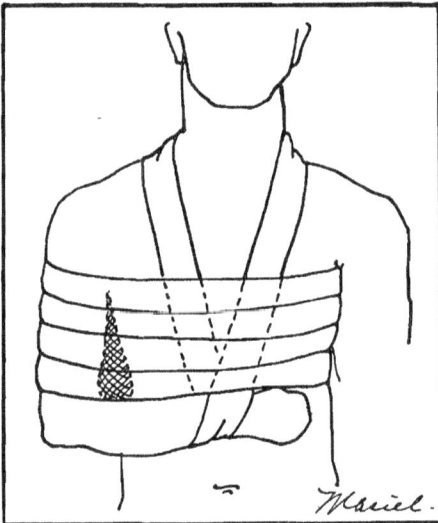

FIG. 14. Dressing for fracture of upper portion of humerus. Donald Gordon. *Am. J. Surg.* New Series, 38, 3, 495, Dec. 1937.

to the side by a swathe of muslin or adhesive plaster, and the forearm supported by a sling with the elbow held at a right angle (Fig. 14). While this arrangement does not insure complete immobilization of the shoulder joint, it does restrict movement sufficiently to prevent displacement *except when the fragments are very oblique.* Many surgeons, however, are apprehensive that the prolonged immobilization with the deltoid muscle stretched and inactive will result in prolonged or occasionally permanent impairment in abduction of the arm. In our experience, and that of others, this fear is not justified and this method is certainly less confining and onerous than when more extensive apparatus is applied.

When the fracture is oblique or reduction cannot be maintained with the arm at the side, some form of abduction splint must be applied. The common ones in use are the aeroplane splint and a shoulder spica with the arm abducted from 45° to 90° (Figs. 16 & 17). These devices are cumbersome, cannot often be worn with clothing and, since many of these patients are obese or senile, the apparatus is difficult to apply or maintain with any degree of comfort to the patient. By some surgeons, they are applied routinely to prevent the deltoid disability referred to above.

When the fracture cannot be reduced by manipulation, continuous traction laterally at a suitable angle should be given a trial. This requires that the patient shall be put to bed under a

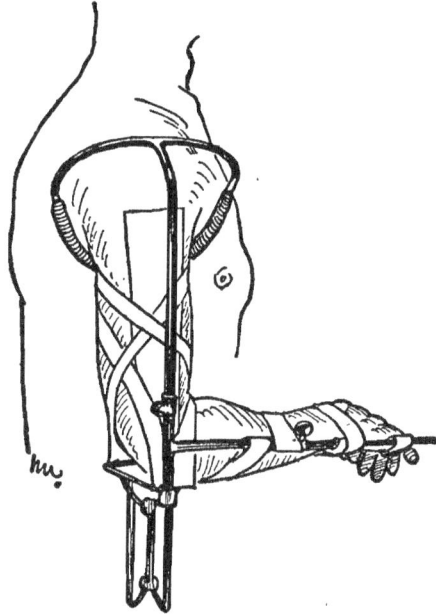

FIG. 15. Jones humerus traction splint. Usually employed only as a temporary dressing. Courtesy of Zimmer Manufacturing Co.

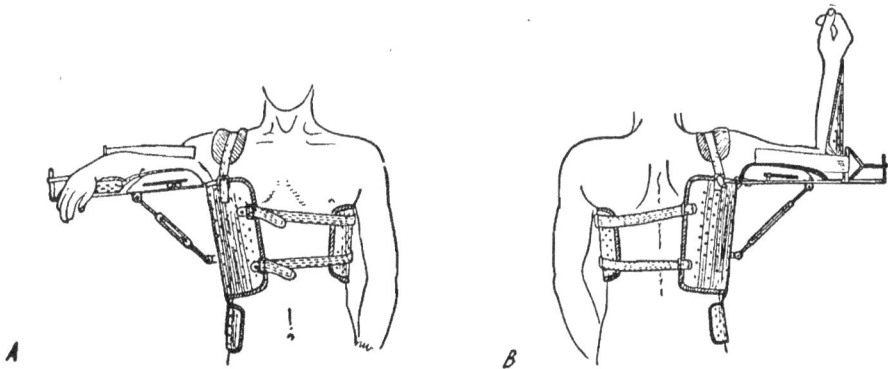

FIG. 16. Type of aeroplane. a) Front view. Arm rotated inward. b) Rear view. Arm rotated outward. Courtesy of Zimmer Manufacturing Co.

Balkan frame (Fig. 19). A Thomas splint is slipped over the arm and the forearm is flexed to a right angle with the humerus. The splint and arm are suspended and counterbalanced under the frame. Traction may be made by a loop about the forearm, but this is prone to slide out of position and it is also liable to cause uncomfortable constriction of the forearm.

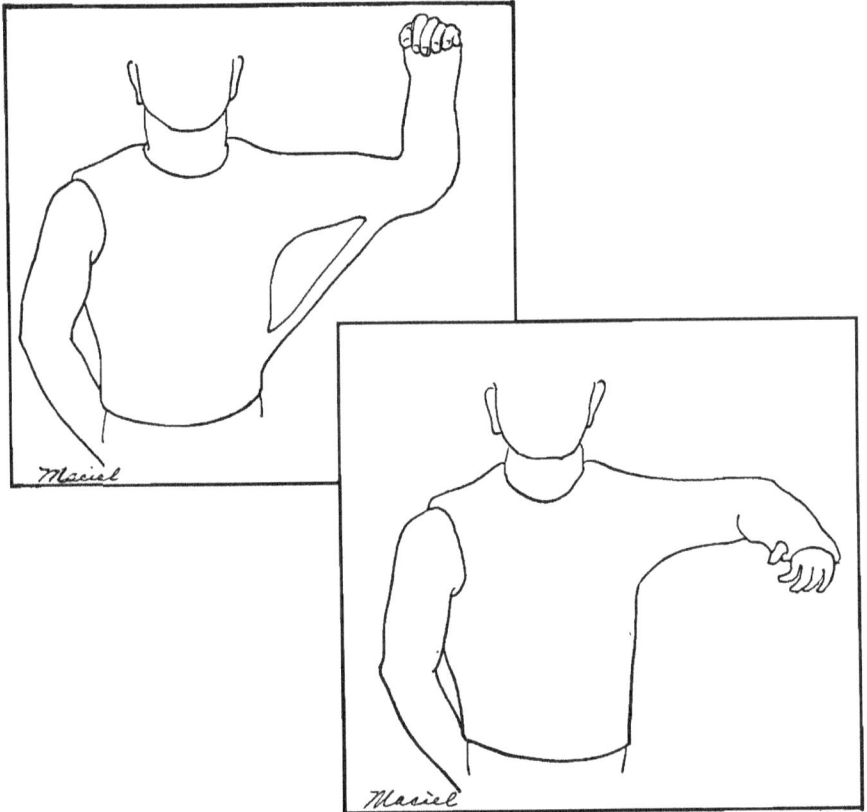

FIG. 17. Two types of shoulder Spica cast. Used when abduction is necessary.

Adhesive plaster to the skin may be used but this is apt to slip, to cause a dermatitis, and it loses much of its effect on the joint by stretching the skin over it. The most effective traction can be obtained by a pin or wire through the olecranon (care being taken not to injure the ulnar nerve).

When portable x-rays show that a satisfactory position has followed traction, the position should be maintained for two to three weeks, when one of the other methods of fixation may be substituted. Occasionally an ambulatory method of traction and abduction may be used as in Fig. 15.

When reduction cannot be obtained by any closed method, open reduction should be done and the arm splinted to the side or in abduction as described. An arm splinted to the side need not, as a rule, be held in this position rigidly more than two weeks. At the end of this time, it should be taken out of all confinement, but the sling to the forearm should be maintained. The patient should be instructed to swing the arm to and fro for a number of times, then lean forward till the trunk is parallel with the floor and swing the arm laterally a number of times. With this regimen, all restriction can be dispensed with in six weeks and impairment of deltoid function rarely persists for any extended period.

Fractures and avulsions of the tuberosities often give rise to prolonged disability and pain. The impairment is in abduction and internal rotation.

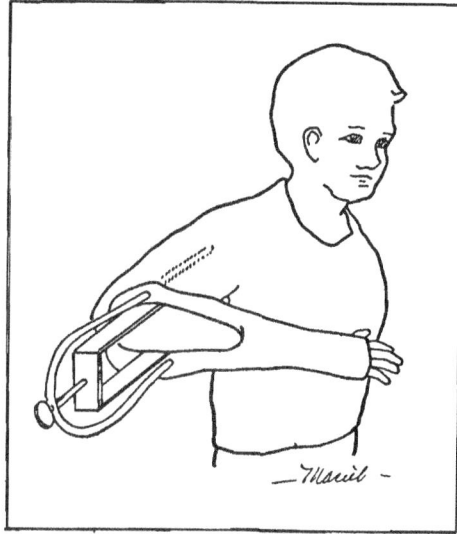

FIG. 18. Hoke apparatus. Used when abduction and traction are necessary and patient can be up.

At first, bed rest with the arm in any comfortable position should be prescribed until acute pain subsides; fixation of the arm to the side by a swathe is often followed by complete settling of the detached fragment into position. The abducted position is uncomfortable and not often necessary. Much of the associated and subsequent pain is due to bursitis which should receive appropriate treatment.

DISLOCATION OF THE HEAD OF THE HUMERUS

VARIETIES

A. Anterior.
  1. Subcoracoid.
  2. Subclavicular.
  3. Subglenoid.
B. Posterior.
C. Inferior-subglenoid.

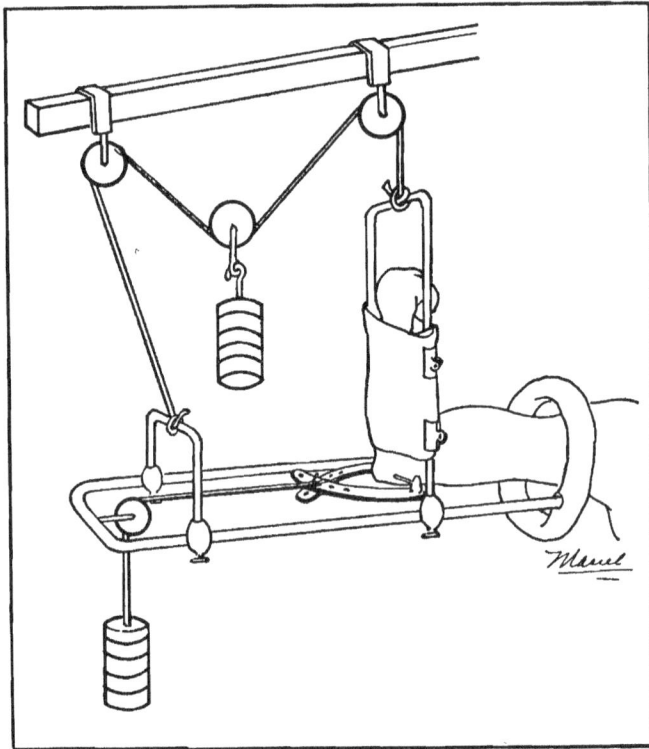

FIG. 19. Traction on humerus by means of Steinman pin through olecranon. Suspended in a Thomas splint. Used when traction is necessary to reduce or hold fragments and patient can not be up and about. Caldwell, John A. and Smith, Josiah. *Am. J. Surg.* New Series, 36: 141-144, Jan. 1936.

CAUSES

Anterior dislocations result from hyperabduction because of falls on the outstretched arm or elbow or direct falls on the shoulder. Posterior dislocations come from falls on the flexed elbow while the arm is abducted and internally rotated.

DIAGNOSIS

A. The pain is of a dull, sickening character as distinguished from the sharp pain of a fracture. There is often considerable shock associated with a dislocation.

B. The shoulder is flattened.

C. The acromion is prominent.

D. The glenoid cavity is empty.

E. The head of the humerus is felt in an abnormal position and rotates with the shaft (unless there is an associated fracture of the neck of the humerus).

F. The axis of the humerus is altered because of the head being displaced medially. When the axis of the humerus is dislocated, the prolonged axis of the humerus passes through the eye on the same side (Fig. 20). Normally it passes two inches lateral to the side of the head.

G. *Dugas sign:* the elbow cannot be placed against the chest when the hand is placed on the opposite shoulder, or conversely when the elbow is held against the chest wall, the hand cannot be placed on the opposite shoulder.

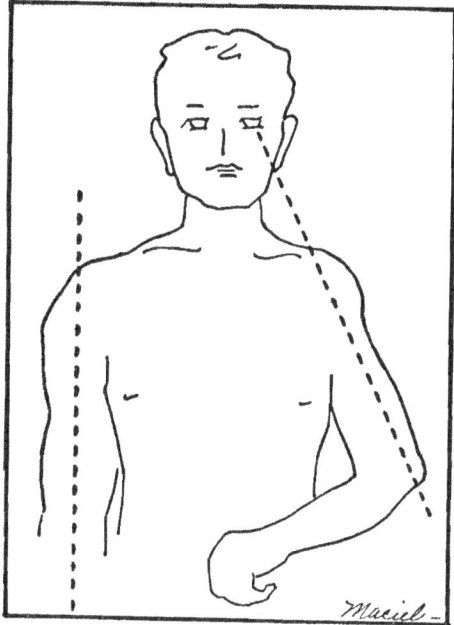

FIG. 20. Anterior dislocation of humerus. Left shoulder is flattened. Axis of humerus when prolonged passes through patient's eye. Normally passes 2 inches outside of patient's head.

REDUCTION

The purpose in all methods of reduction is to make the head traverse the path which it took in dislocating and to pass back through the rent in the capsule. As a rule, complete relaxing anesthesia is necessary and this is best obtained through the use of ether, chloroform, evipal or pentothal sodium. Local anesthesia is often ineffective. If used, it should only be employed by one familiar with its uses. Nitrous oxide is not a good anesthetic for the reason that its use does not accomplish good muscular relaxation. If an attempt is made to reduce without anesthesia, no method should be employed which uses the shaft of the humerus as a lever to overcome the resistance of the engaged head. Fracture of the neck of the humerus may result from trying to pry the head into place with the shaft. It frequently happens that a dislocated head which cannot be moved while the patient is awake and resisting, will fall into place with the slightest manipulations by its own weight as soon as muscular resistance is withdrawn by anesthesia.

Many methods of reduction have been described. The following three are in most common use:

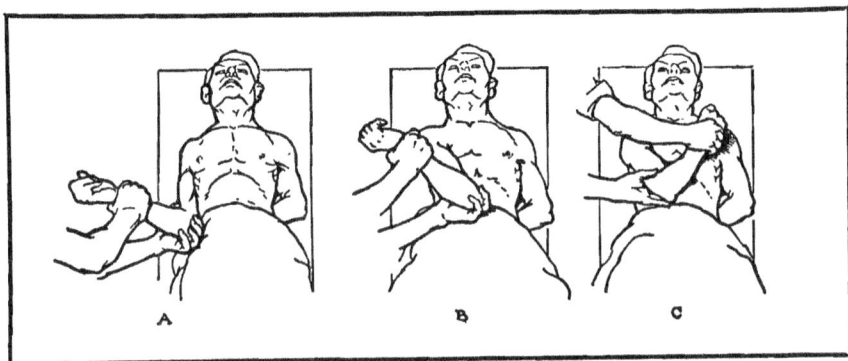

FIG. 21. Kocher Method of reducing subcoracoid dislocation. A, B and C show first, second and third steps. From Homan's *Textbook of Surgery.* Courtesy of Charles C Thomas.

A. *Kocher's method* (Fig. 21), which consists of the following manipulations:

1. Flex the elbow to a right angle.
2. Rotate the arm outward, using the forearm as a lever.
3. Sweep the elbow across the chest.
4. Rotate the arm inward placing the hand on the opposite shoulder.

B. *Traction method.* Traction is made with the arm abducted to a right angle, counter traction being made by the operator placing his unshod heel in the patient's axilla. After a few minutes pull to tire out the patient's resistance, an assistant manipulates the head into position. *Caution:* This is NOT the method where the operator pulls downward with his heel in the axilla and uses his heel as a fulcrum to adduct the arm. *This method is dangerous* and may result in a fracture of the neck of the humerus.

C. *Stimson's method:* The patient is placed in a hammock with a hole in it and the arm hangs through the hole. A weight (10-15 lbs.) is hung on the wrist and in time the resistance of the muscles is overcome and reduction follows spontaneously.

After treatment, the arm should be bandaged to the side of the body for ten days, after this period the forearm should be carried in a sling for four weeks. Complete use should not be resumed in less than six weeks and then all movements of the arm overhead and strain in any direction should be avoided. With each escape of the head from its capsule, subsequent dislocations become easier until the state known as recurrent dislocation is established. In this, the dislocation recurs with but slight stress. This condition is common among epileptics. It requires for its correction some form of operative repair of the capsule and other measures to prevent the head from slipping from the glenoid cavity.

When a dislocation of the head of the humerus has been unreduced for more than six weeks, reduction by manipulation is apt to be unsuccessful. Such conditions should be corrected by open operation. Forceful manipulation in ancient dislocations has resulted in fracture of the neck of the humerus and also tearing of the axillary artery and damage to the brachial plexus. *When reduction is not possible with open operation, the most useful function of the shoulder joint is obtained by resection of the head of the humerus.*

FRACTURES OF SHAFT OF HUMERUS

These occur in any part from the surgical neck to the condyles, and may be due to direct or indirect violence or muscular action. They are often oblique or spiral.

Displacement is not of a constant type but, when the break occurs below the surgical neck and above the insertion of the pectoralis major, the lower fragment is apt to be adducted toward the axilla by the action of the pectoralis major and latissimus dorsi and teres major. When the break is near, but below the insertion of the deltoid muscle, the upper fragment is frequently abducted.

TREATMENT

When the break is above the insertion of the pectoralis major, attempts at reduction should be made under general or local anesthesia. If this is successful, a swathe about the body with the forearm in a sling and with the elbow flexed to a right angle is the simplest dressing and will usually give sufficient fixation (Fig. 14). When reduction is not possible or the break is oblique or comminuted, traction on the humerus with the bone abducted to 45° or less by means of a pin through the olecranon may overcome overriding and permit alignment of fragments (Fig. 19). When this is done, the forearm should be flexed to a right angle to relax the biceps and the arm should be suspended and counterbalanced. After two to three weeks, the patient may be permitted to get up, with a swathe holding the arm to the side. *Early active movements by swinging should be instituted to prevent atrophy of the deltoid muscle.*

When the break is below the insertion of the pectoralis major, one of the following methods may be suitable:

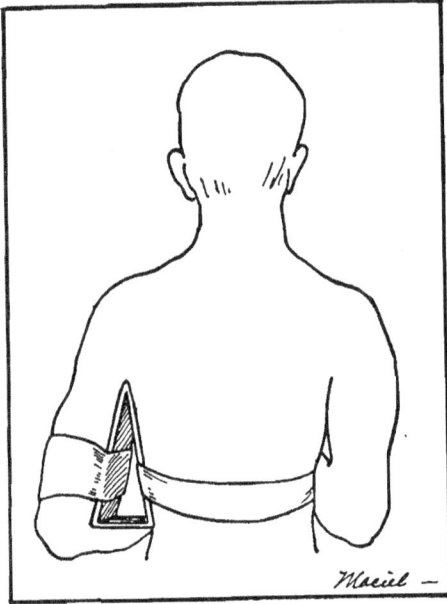

FIG. 22. Mitteldorph triangle. Used when fracture is below insertion of deltoid muscle and some abduction of lower fragment is necessary. Note that triangle does not extend below the bend of the elbow.

1. The fragments may be reduced, and the shoulder and arm and forearm immobilized in a plaster spica with the arm abducted to a suitable angle, usually 45° to 90° (Fig. 17).

2. After a reduction a Mittledorph triangle may be placed between the arm and the chest, and the arm bandaged to this which in turn is strapped to the side (Fig. 22). In fashioning the triangle, care should be exercised that it does not come below the band of the elbow, in order that the forearm may come below it and across the chest.

3. A plaster cast may be applied from axilla to wrist with the elbow flexed to a right angle and the forearm is suspended by a sling passing through a ring incorporated in the cast at the wrist (Fig. 23). The purpose of this dressing is to furnish immobilization of the elbow and coaptation of fragments as well as to make some traction by the weight of the cast. The sling is passed through the ring at the wrist to keep it from being moved toward the elbow and so preventing traction by the cast. In many

cases the patient will have a shorter, more comfortable convalescence and be spared the harassment of a cumbersome dressing if the fracture is exposed and the fragments are reduced and fixed.

When the break is below the insertion of the deltoid muscle, an occasional complication is injury of the radial nerve. This nerve may be severed, contused, pinched, or lacerated at the time of fracture or late paralysis may follow incarceration of the nerve in callus. The symptoms are loss of extensor power of the wrist (wrist drop) and inability to abduct the thumb. *Symptoms of radial nerve paralysis should always be sought at the first examination.*

Radial nerve involvement calls for exploration of the nerve and open fixation of fragments in our opinion. Undoubtedly many of the nerve injuries will recover if treated expect-

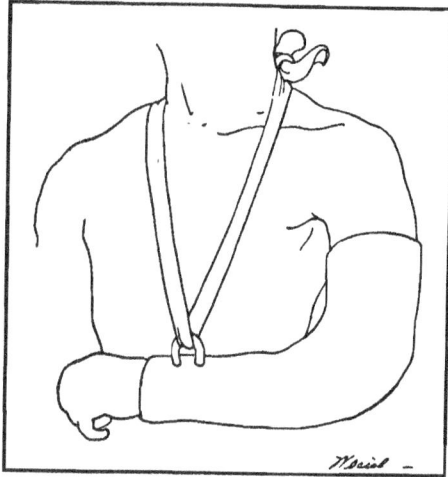

FIG. 23. Hanging cast. Sling is passed through ring embedded in cast at wrist so that sling cannot be slipped toward elbow. Caldwell, John A. *Surg., Gynec. & Obst.*, 70, 421-425. Feb. 15, 1940.

antly, but it is impossible in most instances to determine if the nerve is simply pinched or contused, or if it is severed. An exploration not only settles this question but permits accurate fixation of the fragments and simpler after treatment.

REFERENCES

BUNNELL, S.: Fascial Graft for Dislocation of Acromio Clavicular Joint. *Surg., Gynec. & Obst.*, 46: 563, April 1928.

CALDWELL, JOHN A.: Treatment of Fractures of the Shaft of the Humerus by Hanging Cast. *Surg., Gynec. & Obst.*, 70: 421-425, Feb. 15, 1940.

CODMAN, E. A.: *The Shoulder*. Boston, Thomas Todd Co., 1934.

COTTON, F. J.: *Dislocations and Joint Fractures*. Philadelphia, W. B. Saunders & Co., 1924.

FINDLAY, ROBERT T.: Fractures of the Scapula and Ribs. *Am. J. Surg. New Series*, 38, 3: 489, Dec. 1937.

GRISWOLD, R. A., GOLDBERG, H., and JOPLIN, R.: Fractures of the Humerus. *Am. J. Surg.*, 43: 31, 1939.

LA FERTE, A. D., and ROSENBAUM, M. G.: The "Hanging Cast" in the Treatment of Fractures of the Humerus. *Surg., Gynec. & Obst.*, 65: 231, 1937.

GUNN, MOSES: *Chicago M. J. & Examiner*, 48: 449, 1884.

GURD, FRASER B.: A Simple Effective Method for Treatment of Fractures of the Upper Two-Thirds of the Humerus. *Am. J. Surg.* 47, 2: 443, Feb. 1940.

ROBERTS, S. M.: Fractures of Upper End of Humerus—Advantage of Early Active Motion. *J. A. M. A.*, 98: 367, Jan. 3, 1932.

MEYERDING, H. W.: Treatment of Acromio Clavicular Dislocation. *Surg. Clin. North America*, 17: 1199, 1937.

SCHNEIDER, C. C.: Acromio-Clavicular Dislocation Autoplastic Reconstruction. *J. Bone & Joint Surg.*, 15: 957, Oct. 1933.

SCUDDER, CHARLES L.: *Treatment of Fractures*. Philadelphia, W. B. Saunders Co., Eleventh Ed., 1935.

SPEED, KELLOGG: *Fractures and Dislocations*. Philadelphia, Lea & Febiger, 1935.

WILSON, P. D. and COCHRANE, WM. A.: *Fractures and Dislocations*, Philadelphia, J. B. Lippincott & Co., 1928.

WILSON, PHILIP D.: *Management of Fractures and Dislocations*. Fracture and Dislocations of the Greater Tuberosity of the Humerus, p. 304. Philadelphia, J. B. Lippincott & Co., 1938.

Chapter VI

FRACTURES AND DISLOCATIONS ABOUT ELBOW JOINT

FRACTURE OF THE LOWER END OF THE HUMERUS

The injuries to the lower end of the humerus near the elbow joint will be one of the following (Fig. 24).

1. Supracondylar fracture.
2. Separation of the lower epiphysis.
3. T or Y fractures or more complex forms of comminution.
4. External condyle.

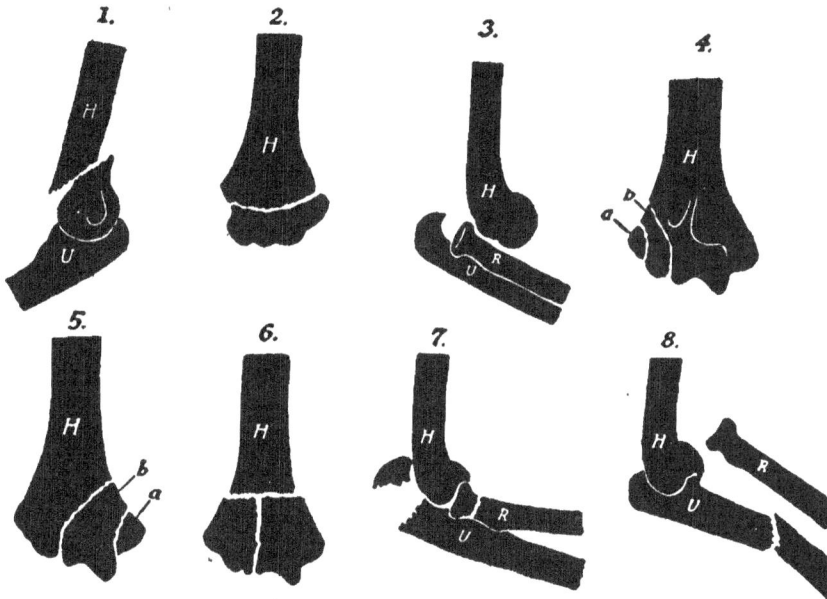

FIG. 24. Commoner fractures about the elbow joint. See illustration Keen's *Surgery*, page 182. Courtesy of W. B. Saunders Co.

5. External epicondyle.
6. Internal condyle.
7. Internal epicondyle.

These fractures must be differentiated from these other conditions about the elbow joint:

1. Fracture of the olecranon.
2. Disclocation of the head of the radius.
3. Dislocation of the elbow (a) lateral, (b) medial, (c) anterior, (d) posterior.
4. Fracture of the head of the radius.

Examination of the Injured Elbow:

1. Normally when the elbow is extended, the three bony prominences—the olecranon, the external and internal condyles are in line. *A departure from this alignment is extremely significant when observed,* but diffuse swelling of the elbow usually obscures the three prominences.

2. Point tenderness should be sought over each of the three prominences as well as the head of the radius.

3. *Gentle attempts* should be made to elicit pain and crepitation on pronation and supination of the forearm.

4. Stimson's sign is elicited by pressure in the long axis of the forearm.

As a rule the only positive diagnosis that can be made is "a swollen elbow" until x-ray films are obtained.

GENERAL CONSIDERATION OF INJURIES ABOUT THE ELBOW JOINT

All fractures about and into the elbow joint are soon followed by great swelling which is due to both ecchymosis into soft tissues and effusion into the joint. This swelling not only prevents accurate diagnosis, but may delay the reduction and treatment most favorable to early restoration. Practically all elbow joint injuries are best treated by fixation in acute flexion, but this position often constricts circulation perilously. Whenever an injured elbow is flexed to an acute angle, the radial pulse *on that side* should be examined. If pulsation cannot be felt or if it is much feebler than *the other one,* the angle of flexion should be increased until the artery is felt beating fully. If the swelling is so great that reduction and right angle fixation is not possible, it is best to put the patient to bed and suspend the arm by the wrist perpendicular to the plane of the body until swelling has subsided. When extreme swelling has developed rapidly, an incision to release imprisoned blood may save some time and reduce chances of infiltration of muscles with venous blood. The best place for the opening is to the outer side of the arm upward from the external condyle. *One of the most dreaded complica-*

tions of fractures about the elbow follows constriction of the circulation after fracture or dislocation and consequent infiltration of the muscles of the forearm by venous blood. The obstruction to circulation may be by too acute flexion of the elbow, or by tight dressing, or a cast. When the muscles become impregnated with venous blood, organization of the blood follows. This, in turn, is followed by fibrosis. By this process the contractile muscle is converted into a fibrous cord with no contractile power. A deformity of the hand follows, in which the fingers are partially flexed, thus resembling a claw. To extend the fingers the wrist must be flexed (Fig. 25). This condition known as Volkmann's contracture (ischaemic paralysis or neuromuscular fibro-

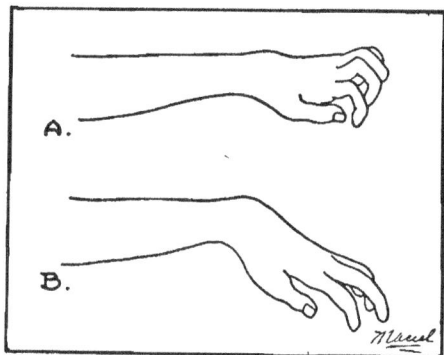

FIG. 25. Volkmann's contracture. a) Typical "claw hand" when wrist is extended. b) When wrist is flexed, fingers can be extended.

sis), is permanent and constitutes a serious impairment and deformity. The cause is organization and fibrosis of muscle engorged with venous blood, and not involvement of any of the peripheral nerves. (The rationale of development of Volkmann's paralysis has been completely and convincingly described by Barney Brooks.)

SUPRACONDYLAR FRACTURES OF THE HUMERUS

This injury is usually seen in children. Clinically, it cannot be distinguished from slipping of the lower epiphysis of the humerus and a separation of the epiphysis is often combined with a fracture of the bone.

The injury is received by falls upon the hand *when the elbow is partially flexed*. When viewed before the quickly supervening swelling masks all deformity, the displaced fragment is seen to project posteriorly and is sometimes displaced laterally also. Point tenderness and Stimson's sign are elicited and manipulation may be associated with crepitus.

Reduction should be attempted as soon as possible. Anesthesia should be complete. Local anesthesia is, in most instances, quite successful and is the most desirable method since attempts at reduction are often unsuccessful and must be repeated.

REDUCTION

The arm is grasped just above the elbow in the operator's left hand and, with the right hand grasping the wrist, the elbow is hyperextended and, *at the same time*, strong traction is made. While the traction is continued, the elbow is flexed to as an acute angle as possible. Before fixing the elbow in acute flexion, the radial pulse should be examined and, if found palpable, the elbow may be fixed in this position. If the radial

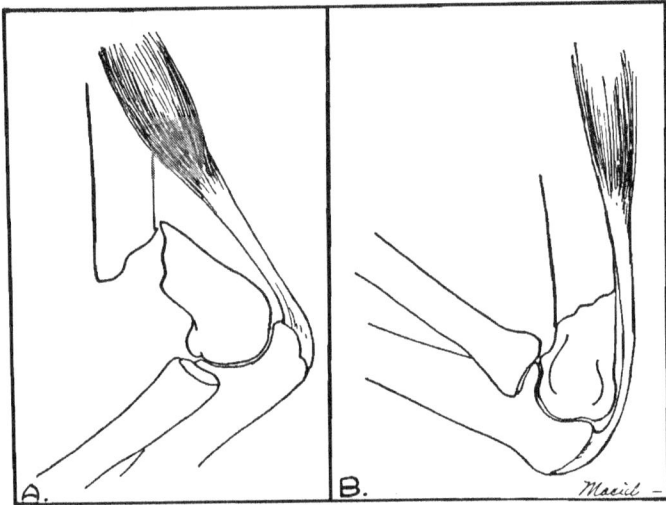

FIG. 26. Supracondylar fracture of humerus. Showing how fracture is reduced by hyperextension followed by flexion while traction is continued and how reduction is held by the tension of the triceps tendon. Adapted from A. P. C. Ashurst's *Fracture of Lower End of Humerus*. Lea & Febiger, 1910.

pulse cannot be felt, the elbow should not be fixed in this position. When the swelling about the elbow has progressed to such degree that sufficient flexion cannot be made to maintain reduction, the arm should be suspended in a posterior splint which holds the elbow slightly flexed and extends beyond the hand. The patient should lie flat and the arm should hang perpendicular.

When reduction is effected, the position is maintained by the tense triceps tendon, drawing the lower fragment upward and preventing the displacement posteriorly, while the coronoid process and soft structures in the cubital fossa press the upper fragment and prevent its forward displacement (Fig. 26).

The effectiveness of the position of acute flexion for maintaining reduction was shown by Hugh Owen Thomas and, later, by Sir Robert
Jones and is often called the Jones position. The decision must be made
as to what method to use to
maintain this position. *Four
methods are in common use:*

1. An encircling cast. This
is certain and not easily disarranged, but extreme care
must be used not to put it on
tight or until swelling has
reached its maximum. An objection is its weight. A
molded posterior plaster
splint answers the same purpose and weighs less than half
as much.

2. Thomas' gage halter.

3. Jones dressing. This is
apt to constrict uncomfortably
(Fig. 27).

4. An Ashhurst dressing
which is the most comfortable
and at the same time quite
effective.

The position of acute flexion should be maintained for

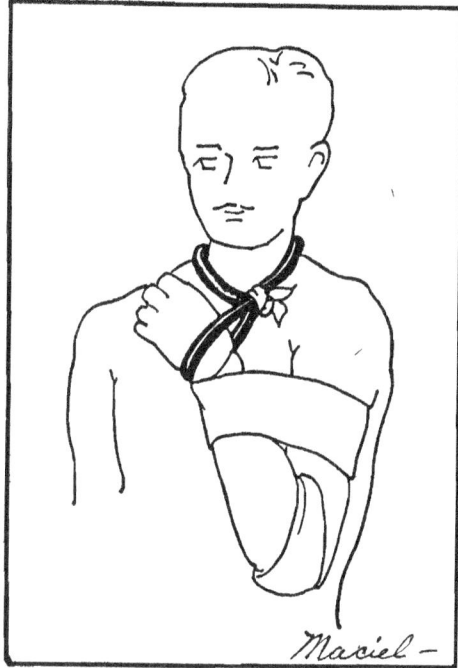

FIG. 27. Jones dressing for supracondylar fracture of humerus. A modification of the "Gage
Halter" of Hugh Owen Thomas.

four weeks when the forearm should be lowered until the elbow is at a
right angle, in which position it is carried in a sling. The arm should be
seen every two or three days, and the angle changed. All dressings can
be removed in six weeks.

Reduction of range of motion is the rule at first but this gradually
increases *with use*. Occasionally, the last 5° to 15° of extension will not
be regained but this diminution causes practically no impairment of
function.

When restricted motion persists, the best means to restore complete
range are baking, massage and passive motion with active exercises.
Forceful manipulation under anesthesia is not only associated with the

danger of producing a fracture, but is followed by such pain and soreness that the joint cannot be moved for some days, and when the discomfort has worn off, the original restriction is present.

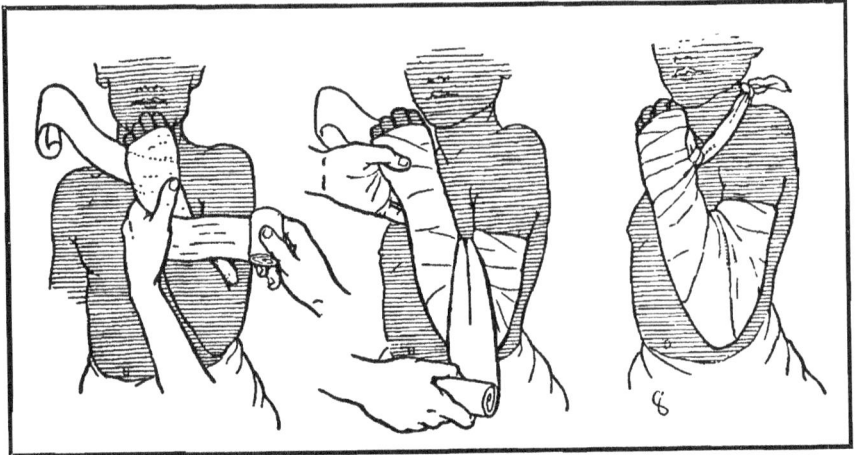

Fig. 28. Hyperflexion bandage of Ashurst. From Homan's *Textbook of Surgery.* Courtesy of Charles C Thomas.

Reasons for the Flexed Position of the Elbow in Fractures About That Joint

1. In supracondylar fractures that position is most favorable for maintaining reduction. In the other fractures, it is quite as satisfactory and relaxes the muscles of the forearm.

2. When splints are removed, gravity aids in restoring extension and greater use of the forearm can be had with the elbow partially flexed which will aid in restoring motion.

3. If ankylosis of the elbow should follow, the arm is most useful at 90° to 100° (the feeding angle). An elbow ankylosed in extension constitutes a severe impairment.

Fractures of the condyles of the humerus, when not greatly displaced, should be treated by flexion. When greatly displaced and restoration by manipulation is not possible, two courses are open:

1. Open Fixation. *This should always be done in children,* especially the inner condyle on account of the possibility of the ulnar nerve being compressed or included in callus.

2. Removal. In adults, when the fragment is small, removal is fol-

lowed by the shorter convalescence. When the fragment is large and extends into the joint, fixation offers the greater chance of use without impairment.

"T" fractures, or those with greater comminution can usually be best treated by one of *three methods:*

1. Molding and reduction under the fluoroscope, and fixation at a right angle by a plaster splint, usually posterior. When this is not possible, the following method may be tried:

2. A pin or wire is passed through the olecranon and the arm is counterbalanced in a Thomas splint under a Balkan frame (Fig. 19). Traction is made by weight attached to the pin or wire.

3. Open operation and fixation is necessary in many cases. *Caution: This procedure is most difficult* and should only be attempted by one with considerable experience.

FRACTURE OF THE OLECRANON

This fracture results from falls on the elbow or blows on that prominence.

The triceps tendon usually pulls the olecranon process up from the shaft of the bone and the separation between the two fragments can be seen or felt. Power of extension of the forearm against gravity or resistance is abolished. Occasionally, this fracture will occur without separation of fragments or tearing of the lateral expansion of the triceps. Such fractures show only pain and swelling and can be diagnosed only by x-ray.

TREATMENT

When fragments are not separated, a sling with elbow joint held at a right angle is the only fixation necessary. *Gentle use* can be started in four weeks and function is usually complete in six to eight weeks.

When fragments are separated and extensor power is gone, *the only proper treatment* is open fixation. The fragment is united to the ulna by wire, catgut, kangaroo tendon, or heavy silk and the tear in the triceps tendon is repaired.

The elbow is fixed at a right angle and gentle use is resumed in two weeks and complete use in six weeks.

The usual treatment to splint fractures of the olecranon in extension is, we believe, extremely bad practice. At least six weeks fixation is necessary, after which restoration of flexion is tedious and painful. This treatment originated when open operation was used only as a last resort. With modern technique and asepsis, there is no reason for considering treatment in extension.

FRACTURE OF THE HEAD AND NECK OF THE RADIUS (FIG. 29 a)

This injury is caused by falls on the outstretched hand.

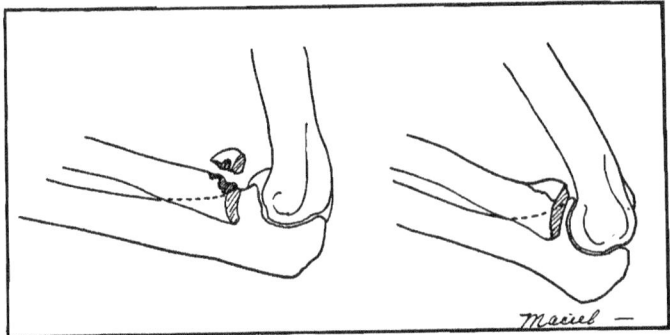

A

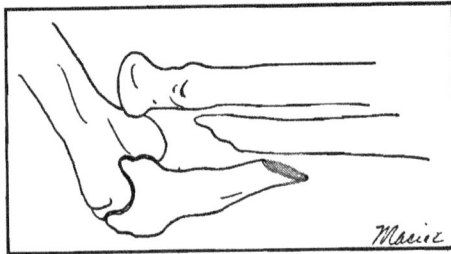

B

FIG. 29. a) Fracture of head of radius. Showing occasional replacement by hyperflexion of elbow. b) Fracture of upper end of ulna with dislocation of head of radius. Monteggia Fracture.

Symptoms

The elbow is swollen most noticeably *on the outer side.*

Pronation and supination cause pain in the region of the head of the radius. This movement may elicit crepitus. X-ray may show the head of the radius cracked or comminuted with fragments displaced to some distance. Occasionally, a completely detached head may be turned or reversed, or displaced to some distance.

TREATMENT

Cracks without displacement may be treated conservatively by a sling with the elbow at a right angle and a splint to prevent rotation of the forearm. A detached or comminuted head should be removed by open operation. The incision should be made between the head of the radius and the olecranon. Care should be observed in extending this incision downward lest the posterior interosseous nerve be cut where it passes through the supinator muscle.

Removal of the head is generally to be preferred to attempts to replace fragments. When the displaced pieces unite in good position, there is strong probability that in healing they will adhere to the annular ligament surrounding the head of the bone and so prevent pronation and supination. Removal of the head does not cause great impairment of elbow function or reduce materially range of pronation and supination.

DISLOCATION OF THE ELBOW JOINT

1. Posterior.
2. Anterior.
3. Medial.
4. Lateral.
5. Combined when the radius and ulna separate and the articular surface of the humerus descends between them.
6. Dislocation of the head of the radius.

REDUCTION

1). *Posterior dislocation is by far the most common;* the others are comparatively rare. It is caused by falls on the outstretched hand when the elbow is extended. A common complication is fracture of the coronoid process. On inspection, the elbow is held rigidly flexed, the olecranon projects backward, forming a protuberance at the lower end of the humerus and the forearm appears shortened.

Here again reduction should not be forced but resistance should be relaxed by anesthesia. The forearm should be fully supinated to relax the biceps muscle; it is then fully extended and strongly pulled upon while the forearm is gradually flexed. After reduction, a Schantz dressing is applied with the elbow at a right angle or less.

2). *Anterior dislocation* is produced by forced pronation and hyperextension.

The forearm is supinated and hyperextended, and the head of the radius is forced backward by direct pressure while the forearm is flexed. Dressing is as for posterior dislocation.

3). *Lateral and medial dislocations* are rare and are produced by hyperextension and abduction or adduction. Deformity is evident though fractures must be excluded by x-ray.

Reduction is by hyperextension and traction while the elbow is pressed laterally.

4). Combined dislocation is rare without fracture. The distinguishing deformity is wide spreading of the joint. Reduction and splinting is as follows. The elbow is flexed to ninety degrees and then pulled down while the condyles of the humerus are compressed. The elbow is splinted at ninety degrees with the forearm supinated.

5). Dislocation of the head of the radius is fairly common and results from falls on the extended hand. It is frequently associated with fracture of the ulna in its proximal three or four inches.

The head of the radius is seen projecting in front and to the outer side of the external condyle.

Reduction is accomplished by supinating and hyperextending the forearm and pressing the head of the radius into place—after which the elbow is splinted in acute flexion and supination.

Monteggia Fracture

Anterior dislocation of the head of the radius with fracture of the ulna within its upper third is a combination often described as the Monteggia fracture. The head of the radius may be displaced anteriorly when the fracture of the ulna will be angulated in the same direction. In other cases the ulna may be angulated posteriorly when the head of the radius is extruded through the posterior part of the capsule and appears behind and to the outer side of the joint. Whenever x-ray of the elbow shows a fracture of the ulna a short distance below the joint and the head of the radius in normal position, the Monteggia combination should be suspected. Frequently a later film may show the head of the radius displaced.

These fractures should be reduced by traction and flexion and should be held by a cast with the elbow acutely flexed and the forearm supinated. If reduction is not maintained, open fixation of the elbow with plastic repair of the annular ligament should be carried out—a procedure completely discussed and described by J. S. Speed. In management of this

fracture it should not be forgotten that union is frequently quite delayed in the upper four inches of the ulna.

COMPLICATIONS OF INJURIES ABOUT THE ELBOW

1. Volkmann's contracture has been described and discussed.

2. Injury to the ulnar nerve may occur in fractures of the internal
condyle. It may happen at the time of injury or occur late from incarceration of the nerve in callus. Late ulnar nerve involvement may also
take place following fracture of the external condyle which is not reduced or fixed in place. This fracture permits lateral shifting of the
humeral articulation and consequent stretching of the ulnar nerve.

3. Radial nerve palsy may occur early or late.

4. Medial nerve involvement is rare.

5. "Gun stock deformity" by which is meant lateral angulation of
the elbow joint and alternation of the carrying angle.

6. Some restricted motion for a time is almost constant in all elbow
injuries, but permanent restriction of motion often persists in the form
of failure to completely flex and extend the joint. Ankylosis is not common, except in severe injuries in patients predisposed to arthritic changes.

REFERENCES

ASHHURST, A. P. C.: *Fractures of Lower End of Humerus*. Philadelphia, Lea
& Febiger, 1910.

BÖHLER, LORENZ A.: *Treatment of Fractures*. Fractures of the Shaft of the
Humerus. Baltimore, Wm. Wood & Co., 1935.

BROOKS, BARNEY: Volkmann's Contracture. *Arch. Surg.*, 5: 188.

CALDWELL, JOHN A.: Treatment of Fractures in the Cincinnati General
Hospital. *Ann. Surg.* 97, 2: 172, Feb. 1933.

DUDGEON, L. S.: Volkmann's Contracture. *Lancet*, Jan. 11, 1902.

JONES, ROBERT: Fractures about Elbow Joint. *Provincial M. J.*, 14: 28,
Jan. 1895.

SPEED, KELLOGG: Fracture of Head of Radius. *Am. J. Surg.*, 38: 157, June
1924.

SPEED, J. S. and BOYD, HAROLD B.: Treatment of Fractures of the Ulna with
Dislocation of the Head of the Radius. Monteggia Fracture. *J. A. M. A.*,
CXV, 1699. Nov. 16, 1940.

VAN GORDER, GEO. W.: Surgical Approach in Supra-Condylar T Fractures
of the Humerus Requiring Open Reduction. *J. Bone & Joint Surg.*,
22, 2: 278, Apr. 1940.

VOLKMANN: Ischaemic Paralysis. *Zentralbl. f. Chir.*, 8: 801, 1881.

WILSON, P. D.: Fractures and Dislocations in Region of the Elbow. *Surg.,
Gynec. & Obst.*, 56:335, Feb. 15, 1933.

Chapter VII

FRACTURES OF RADIUS AND ULNA. FRACTURES AND DISLOCATIONS ABOUT WRIST JOINT. FRACTURES AND DISLOCATIONS OF CARPAL BONES AND PHALANGES

FRACTURES of one or both bones of the forearm may occur in any part *but are less frequent in the upper third because of the heavy covering of muscle.* Practically any form of direct or indirect violence may cause the forearm to be broken. At present automobile injuries account for many such fractures. Green-stick fractures are quite common in children.

SYMPTOMS

When *both bones* are broken, free mobility and deformity is evident, and crepitus is easily elicited. When but *one bone* is fractured, mobility must often be sought and point tenderness and Stimson's sign must be elicited. *In green-stick fractures,* extreme bowing without mobility and point tenderness are the predominating signs. Much has been written concerning the direction and type of displacement in fractures in different parts of the forearm and how these displacements should be corrected by position of the limb. Most of the rules to be followed originated from anatomic studies and observation after death and *in days before the x-ray was in use.* Since the x-ray is now in universal use, the type of displacement and optimum position for splinting have been found to be inconstant. The only satisfactory plan is to try to reduce by manipulation and *check by x-ray.* Local anesthesia, if properly carried out, is particularly useful in forearm fractures because manipulation must often be repeated when x-ray check fails to show satisfactory position. When both bones are broken, the local anesthetic must be injected about both fractures.

REDUCTION

The elbow is flexed to a right angle and a wide, well padded sling is thrown about the arm just above the elbow and is fastened to a firm object (bed post) for counter-traction. An assistant grasps the patient's thumb in one hand and his four fingers in the other and makes steady traction in the long axis of the forearm. Painting the fingers with compound tincture of benzoin will prevent them from slipping from the grip of the assistant. Weights or springs may also be used to maintain the pull on the forearm if adequate equipment is available. The operator then manipulates by pronation and supination, and angulation and molding. After reduction is thought to be satisfactory, a cast without padding is applied from axilla to hand. As a rule fractures in the upper third are best splinted in supination, while those lower down are most frequently held in mid-pronation, *but this rule is not invariable.* Rounded wood dowels ⅜" in diameter, pressed into the surface of the plaster over the interosseous space front and back, often force the fragments of the radius and ulna apart and prevent fusion of the two bones in a common mass of callus (Fig. 30).

We have found some form of apparatus which maintains traction and holds the forearm in position while the cast is being applied a great

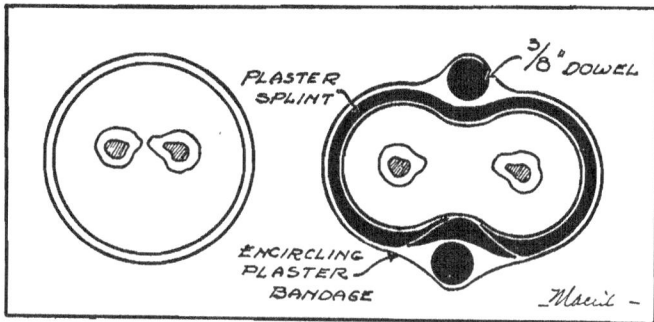

FIG. 30. Fractures of radius and ulna. Showing how fragments of radius and ulna are separated when pieces of wooden dowels are placed on opposite sides of the interosseous space and compressed by encircling plaster bandage. Adapted from Böhler, Lorenz A., *Treatment of Fractures.* Williams & Wilkins. 1936.

help in putting up these fractures. In our clinic the apparatus (Fig. 31) described by the author, in which "finger grips" are used to make the pull on the fingers, has been found most useful; the reduction and traction outfit of Soutter is also excellent.

Good function of the forearm requires that pronation and supination shall be free. This movement is apt to be restricted when reduction is not accurate and union takes place with a considerable mass of callus. For this reason an accurate reduction is important and open fixation should be employed if a good reduction cannot be attained my manipulation. When but one bone can be reduced, effort should be made to get the fragments of the radius in good position rather than the ulna. In ten to fourteen days this bone will be somewhat fixed by provisional callus and the fragments of the ulna can then be put in position by open operation. The reason for this plan is that since the ulna is subcutaneous throughout its course, open operation on it is much easier than on the radius. Any reduction of fracture of both bones should be checked at rather frequent intervals during the first two weeks, since displacement occurs even with the most rigid and effective splinting.

The most serious complication of fracture of the radius and ulna is a

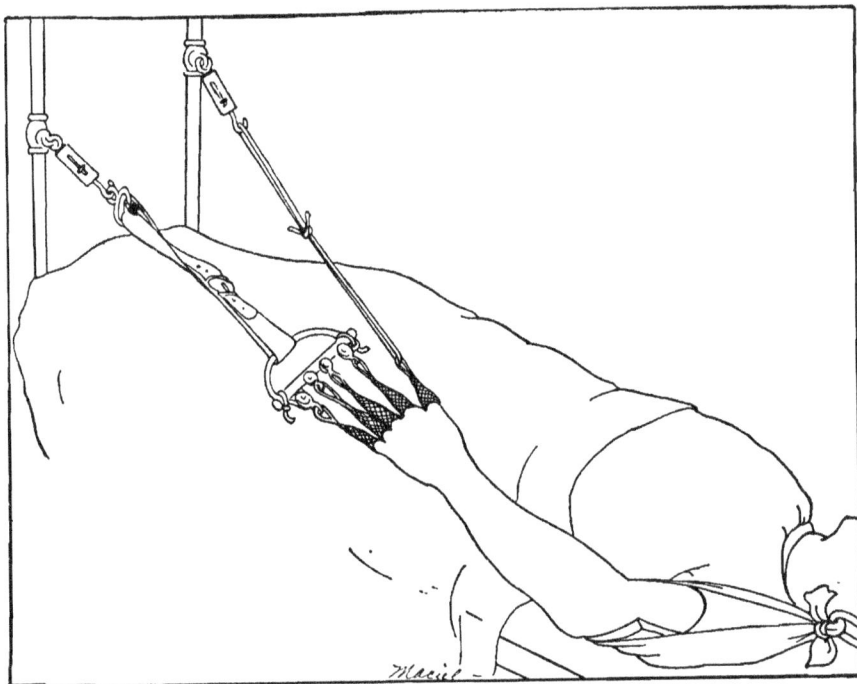

FIG. 31. Reduction of fractures of radius and ulna with traction by means of finger grips. Author's method. Traction and counter traction may be made from standards at opposite ends of fracture table or from head and foot bars on the hospital bed, or by use of the Souttar apparatus.

synostosis between the two bones resulting in abolition of pronation and supination.

Oblique fracture of the radius alone in its lower third is often difficult to reduce and hold on account of the lateral pull of the pronator quadratus. Such breaks should be fixed by open operation if good closed reduction cannot be made.

Splinting should be continued for six to eight weeks. No splint should restrict the use of the fingers but active function of these members should be encouraged during fixation of the forearm.

FRACTURES OF THE LOWER END OF THE FOREARM

These include:

1. Lower end of ulna.
2. Styloid process of the ulna.
3. Colles' fracture.
4. Reverse Colles' fracture.

1. Fracture of *the lower end of the ulna* is sometimes called "parry fracture and thug's fracture" because it is frequently received by the victim raising his arm over his head to "parry" a blow from a club. This fracture is usually evident by all signs. It is not often much displaced and is easily reduced.

The best fixation is a plaster cuff to the elbow leaving the fingers free for use.

2. Fracture of *the ulnar styloid process*. This accident can result from direct injury and also by evulsion from forcible adduction of the wrist. Treatment is splinting in abduction by a palmar splint for two to three weeks.

COLLES' FRACTURE

Colles' fracture receives its name from the Irish surgeon, Abraham Colles, who described this fracture and its mechanism of production in the *Edinburg Medical Journal*, 1814. The break comes about, in the vast majority of cases, by falls on the outstretched hand, the line of force being slightly off the long axis of the forearm. Compression fracture of the wrist is another name which is in common use. When the force is sufficient, the lower end of the radius is impacted and cracked longitudinally if the line is not much off the axis of the forearm. When, as is usually the case, it passes posterior to the radius, the lower fragment is pushed upward and backward and occasionally lies on the dorsal surface of the upper fragment. Frequently the ulnar styloid process is also broken off.

Appearance of the wrist: The entire joint is swollen. If the lower fragment is displaced dorsally, there is a prominence on the dorsum of the wrist just above the joint and the palmar surface below this point is prominent, giving a distinct bend in the wrist at the point of fracture. A lateral view of the wrist shows somewhat the outline of a silver dinner

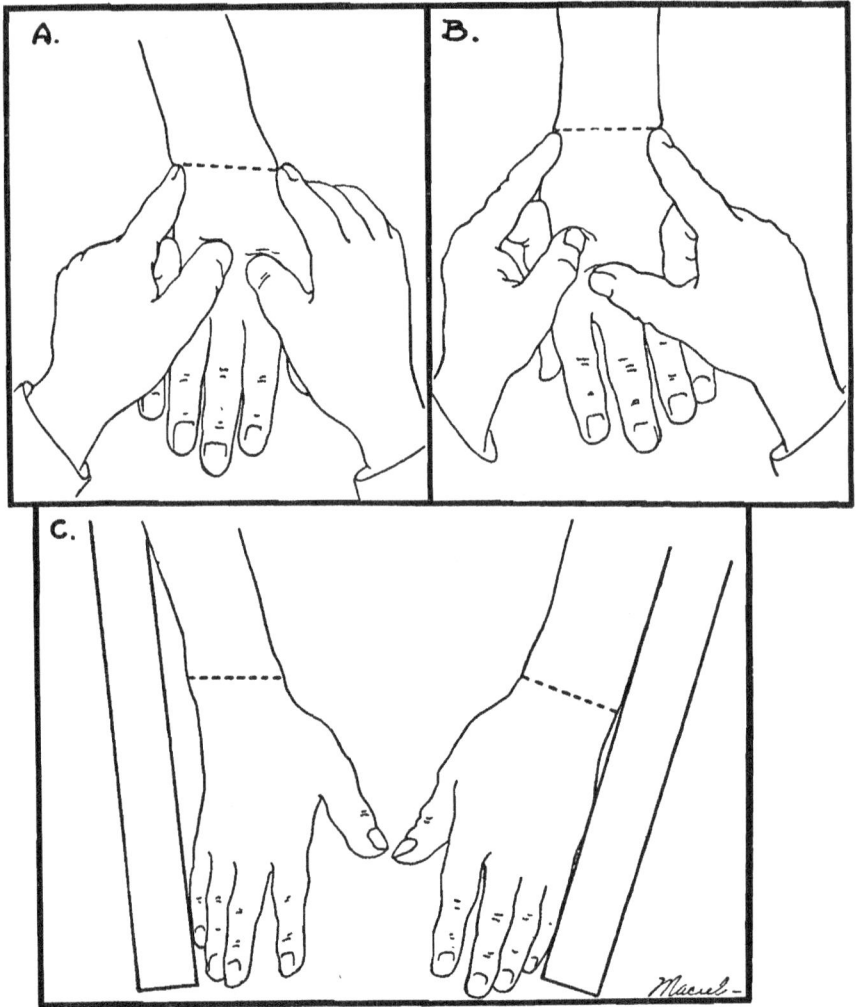

FIG. 32. Colles' fracture. The most common deformity. Drawing up of the radial styloid process. a) Normal relation of the styloid process about ⅜″ distad of the ulnar styloid process. b) In Colles' fracture the radial styloid process is pushed up until it is even with or proximad of the ulnar styloid process. c) Normally a straight edge placed against the outer condyle of the humerus and the little finger misses the ulnar styloid process about ¾″. d) When a Colles' fracture is present, a straight edge touches the ulnar styloid process when placed against the outer condyle of the humerus and the little finger.

fork, hence the common designation "silver fork deformity". This deformity, however, is more frequently absent than present, owing to greater frequency of impaction than displacement of the lower fragment. A more constant deformity is elevation of the radial styloid process, which occurs with either impaction or displacement. Normally, the radial styloid process is ⅜″ distal of the ulnar, and a line drawn between the two inclines downward or distally on the radial side. In Colles' fracture, this line will extend at a right angle to the long axis of the forearm or the radial prominence and may even be the proximal one (Fig. 32, a & b).

On account of the shortening of the radius, the hand will deviate toward the radial side. This can be shown by holding a straight edge in contact with the outer condyle of the humerus and the distal end of the metacarpal of the little finger. Normally, the straight edge will fail to come in contact with the ulnar styloid process by ¾″ (Fig. 32, c & d). In Colles' fracture, it will touch the ulnar styloid process. Point tenderness can be elicited just above the wrist.

REDUCTION

Local anesthesia is nearly always successful if the hematoma can be infiltrated. Strong traction is made on the wrist at the same time hyper-

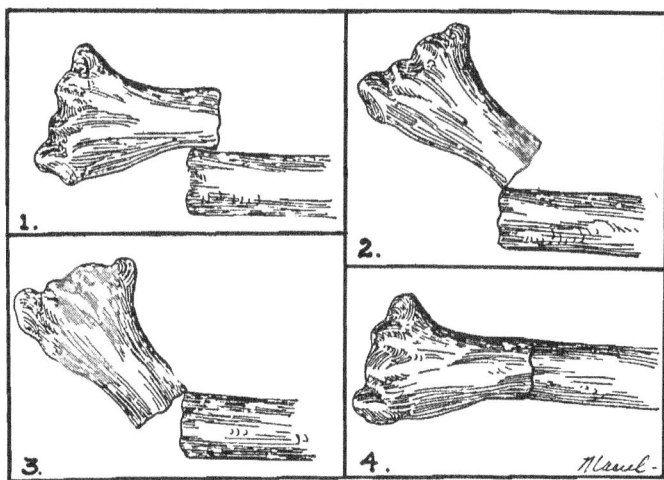

FIG. 33. Diagram showing successive maneuvers for reducing the dorsal displacement in Colles' fracture. 1) Fragment dorsally displaced. 2) Hyperextension of wrist. 3) Traction on wrist with pressure downward. 4) Flexion of wrist.

extending and pulling to the ulnar side. While continuing the extension, the wrist is flexed (Fig. 33). Reduction is maintained during splinting by traction on the thumb with one hand and the fingers with the other by an assistant, the elbow being fixed by a sling about the arm fastened to a fixed post. We have found the finger grip traction outfit described by the author excellent for this purpose. While the arm is held, plaster splints are applied on the front and back of the arm; these extend from the elbow to the distal ends of the metacarpal bones, *never far enough to interfere with the movement of the fingers*. The splints should be wrapped with one or two plaster rolls, and *the entire cast thus formed*

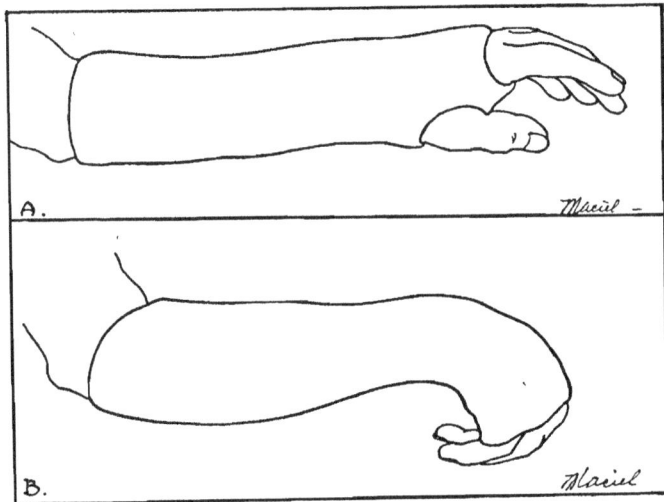

FIG. 34. Dressings for Colles' fracture. a) Hand in position of rest. Encircling plaster from elbow to ends of metacarpals, leaving fingers to move freely. b) When fracture is oblique and difficult to keep in place, this position should be used. It is not comfortable and should be changed to "a" in 10 to 14 days.

should be split on the ulnar side after it has hardened 15 to 30 minutes. The hand should be splinted *in the position of rest* with the wrist slightly extended (Fig. 34a). Occasionally, when the break is very oblique, the wrist must be flexed and deviated to the ulnar side to maintain reduction (Fig. 34b). When this is done, the position should be changed to the more comfortable one of rest in ten days. Otherwise the dressing should not be disturbed for four weeks, during which time the patient should be encouraged to use the hand as much as possible. A check x-ray should show the following points to fulfill requirement for a successful reduction:

1. The relations of the two styloid processes should be normal, i.e., the radial styloid process should be ⅜ to ½″ distal of the ulnar.
2. The ulnar deviation should be corrected.
3. A lateral view should show a line connecting the margins of the

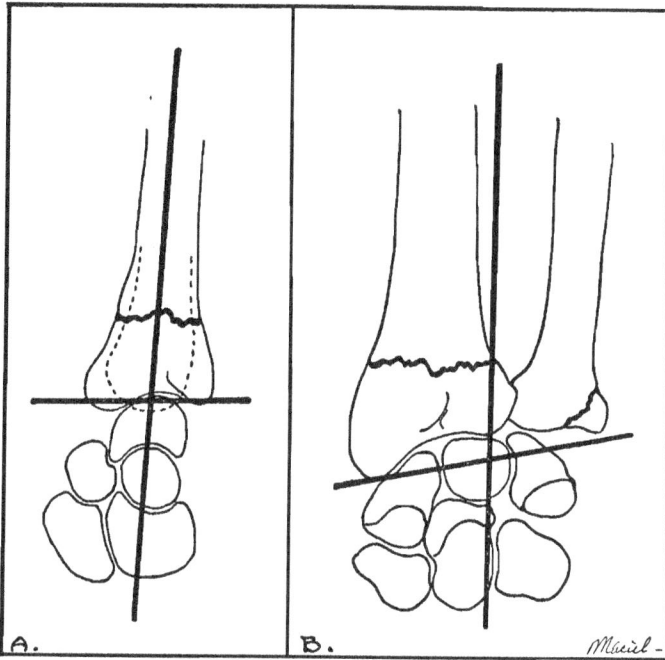

Fig. 35. Tracings from roentgenograms. Well reduced Colles' fracture. a) Lateral view. Line across articular surface at right angle to axis of radius. b) Anteroposterior view. Radial styloid process lower than that of the ulnar. Line joining the two processes not at 90° with the axis of the forearm.

radial articular surface at a right angle to the long axis of the radius Figs. 35 & 36).

REVERSED COLLES' FRACTURE

In this injury, while the fracture is in the lower end of the radius—the distal fragment is displaced onto the palmar surface of the wrist. It is caused by direct violence over the wrist or by falls on the arm with the wrist bent under the body. The anterior displacement of the lower fragment causes a deformity which has been given the name "garden spade".

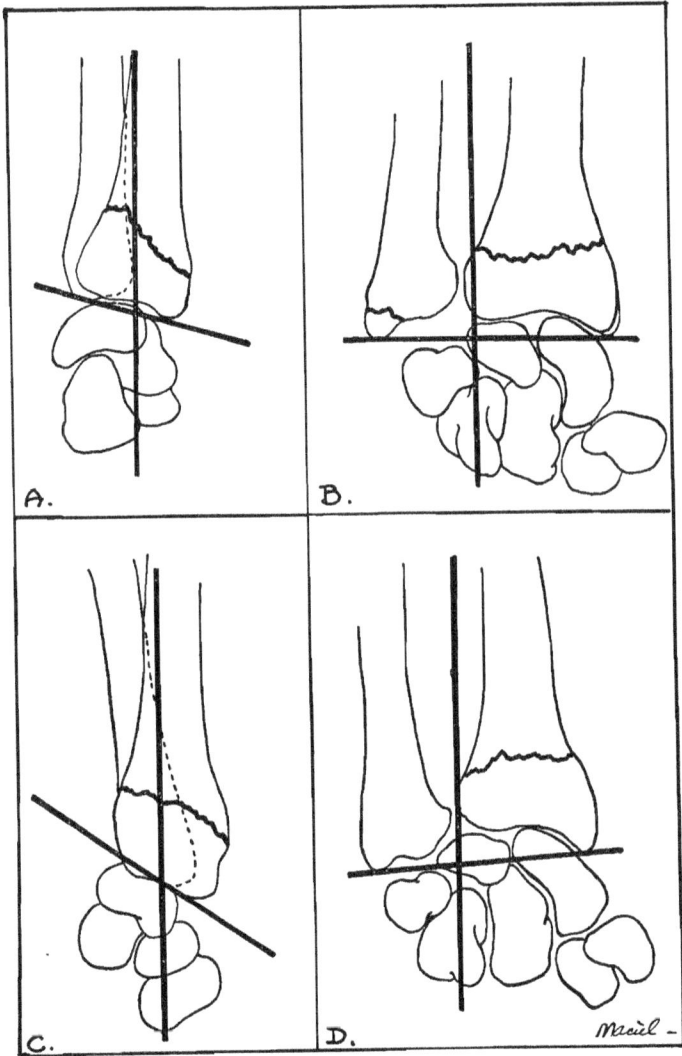

Fig. 36. Tracings from roentgenograms. Incompletely reduced Colles' fracture. a) and c) Lateral views. Lines across articular surfaces not at a right angle to axis of humerus. b) and d) Line joining styloid processes crosses axis of forearm at 90°. Radial styloid process should be ⅜" distad of ulnar.

Reduction is made by extreme flexion of the wrist with traction, then while a strong pull is maintained the wrist is hyperextended. After reduction the forearm should be encased in plaster from the fingers to the mid humerus in the following position: Wrist and hand fully extended (cockup position), wrist supinated—elbow flexed to 90 degrees.

Reduction of this fracture is difficult to accomplish and uncertain to maintain. Many of these breaks require open fixation.

The reverse Colles' is much rarer than the true Colles' fracture. It is unfortunate that the name of Colles is associated with this fracture since it is not caused by compression force—and reduction—treatment and prognosis are all different from the classical Colles' fracture.

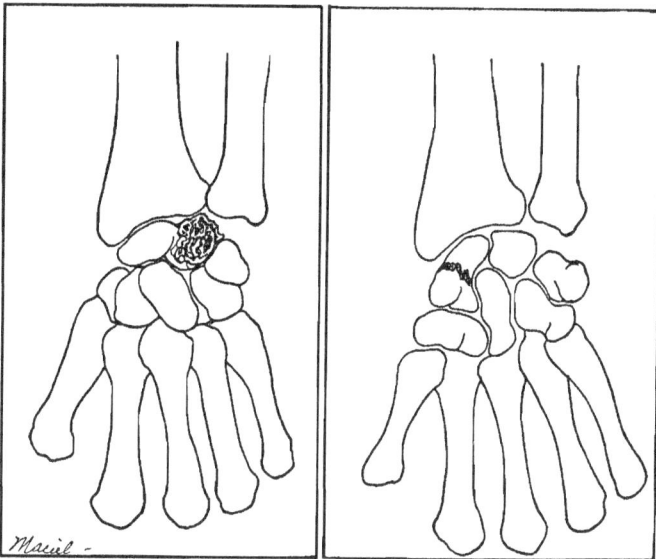

FIG. 37. Fracture of carpal lunate. Often crushed.

FIG. 38. Fracture of carpal navicular. Usually transverse.

FRACTURES OF THE CARPAL BONES

The bones most commonly affected are the lunate (Fig. 37) and navicular (Fig. 38); both are fractured by falls on the outstretched palm. Fracture of the navicular is recognized by tenderness over the bone and on pressure in the tabetiere. The depression of the tabetiere is eliminated.

Fracture of the lunate cannot certainly be diagnosed except by x-ray. Pressure over the palmar and dorsal surfaces of the bone may furnish presumptive evidence.

Fracture of either bone should be treated by splinting the wrist with a plaster gauntlet extending to the elbow, leaving the fingers free. This

should be continued for two to three months. Shorter period of treatment is apt to be followed by prolonged pain in the wrist. Failure of
union in fracture of the navicular is common. Both of these bones are
occasionally dislocated on the palmar surface. Reduction is affected by
extending the wrist and pressing the displaced bone into place while
flexing the wrist. A rounded stick (a short section of broom handle)

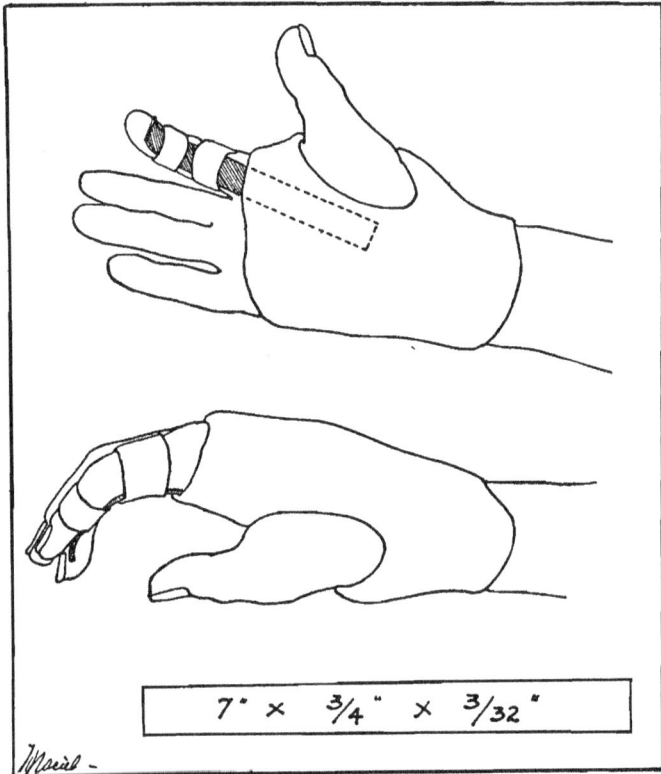

FIG. 39. Method of reducing and splinting a fracture of a phalanx or metacarpal bone.
A cast is applied incorporating the aluminum splint in a straight position. When the
plaster has "set" the finger is pulled upon and strapped tight to the splint after which
finger and splint are bent together to the desired degree of flexion.

is useful for this. When reduction is impossible by manipulation, open
operation is necessary and, when reduction has been delayed, removal
of the displaced bone is often the best treatment.

Fractures of the metacarpal bones result from direct injury and are frequently due to injudicious pugilism. There is diffuse swelling over the dorsum of the hand. Point tenderness over the point of fracture and Stimson's sign are elicited; the last is a most important diagnostic sign in these fractures.

Reduction is by traction on the fingers and manipulation. If accurate reduction is not possible by manipulation, open repair should be done since a synostosis between metacarpal bones may cause some crippling of the fingers. Splinting is best done with molded plaster, either dorsal or palmar, and should include the wrist as well as the finger of the broken metacarpal and be continued for three weeks.

FRACTURE OF THE PHALANGES

Any phalanx may be broken, nearly always by direct violence. All symptoms are usually present, though positive diagnosis is not always

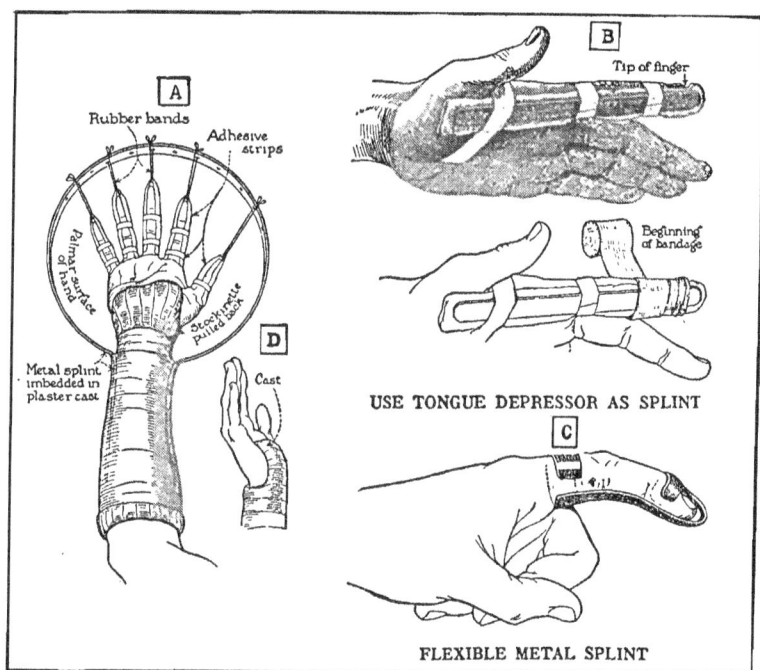

FIG. 40. Methods of splinting fractures of the carpus-metacarpus and phalanges. a) Banjo splint. Traction may be made on fingers by adhesive plaster or pin through phalanges. b) Tongue blade splint for finger. An excellent emergency dressing. Usually too straight for proper position or comfort. From *Primer on Fractures*. Cooperative Committee on Fractures. American Medical Association.

possible except by x-ray. Transverse fractures can nearly always be reduced by manipulation. A number of types of splint are in use:

1. A wooden tongue blade (Fig. 40a). This is often effective for a distal phalanx, but for a middle or proximal phalanx the straight position is uncomfortable.

2. Bandaging the finger over a roller bandage gripped in the hand. This often produces too great flexion and ties up the entire hand.

The best method is by a plaster cast which includes wrist and hand and in this is incorporated an aluminum strip which is as wide as the finger and extends to its end. As soon as the plaster has hardened sufficiently to hold the aluminum strip firmly, the finger is stretched and bandaged firmly to the aluminum, after which finger and splint are bent together to a suitable position (Fig. 39). The maneuver makes sufficient traction to reduce oblique fractures which cannot otherwise be made to engage.

When the fractures are compound or comminuted, some form of traction must be applied. The most suitable device for this is the Banjo splint Fig. 40a). A plaster cast is applied from elbow to wrist and in this is incorporated a loop of iron bar ⅛″ in diameter. This should extend at least three inches beyond the finger and be four inches wider than the hand. Traction is made by means of rubber bands attached to the wire loop and to the fingers by means of adhesive plaster or wires passing through the distal phalanx. As soon as union has started, this dressing should be discontinued and the first device described should be substituted.

DISLOCATIONS OF THE THUMB

These occur at the metacarpophalangeal joint and at the second joint of the thumb and are brought on by hyperextension of the thumb. They are extremely painful, accompanied by much swelling, and are often difficult to reduce.

The dislocation is nearly always posterior, anterior and lateral dislocations being rare. Reduction is by traction and hyperextension (in posterior dislocations) and by flexion in anterior dislocations. Occasionally the displaced articular surface is extruded between the extensor tendons and engaged so firmly that open reduction is necessary. After reduction, the thumb should be splinted in abduction by plaster or a dressing of the Schanz type.

Any phalangeal joint may be dislocated backward, forward or laterally. Reduction is by traction and bending the finger in the direction opposite to the dislocation. Occasionally, repair of the capsule is necessary to prevent recurrence of the displacement.

REFERENCES

BÖHLER, LORENZ A.: *Treatment of Fractures. Fractures of the Radius and Ulna.* New York. Wm. Wood & Co., 1936.

COLLES, ABRAHAM: Colles' Fracture. *Edinburgh M. J.*, 182: April 1814.

CALDWELL, JOHN A.: Device for Making Traction on the Fingers. *J. A. M. A.*, 96: 1226, Apr. 11, 1931.

DAVIS, G. G.: Treatment of Dislocated Semilunar Carpal Bones. *Surg., Gynec. & Obst.*, 37: 225, Aug. 1923.

GURD, FRASER B.: The Colles-Ponteau Fracture of the Lower End of the Radius. *Am. J. Surg. New Series*, 38, 3: 526-538, Dec. 1937.

LEWIS, K. M.: Colles' Fracture. *Ann. Surg.*, 99: 510, March 1934.

RIDER, DEAN L.: Fractures of the Metacarpals—Metatarsals, and Phalanges. *Am. J. Surg. New Series*, 38, 3: 549, Dec. 1937.

SNODGRASS, L. E.: Fractures of the Carpal Bones. *Am. J. Surg. New Series*, 38, 3: 539, Dec. 1937.

SNODGRASS, L. E.: End Results of Carpal Scaphoid Fractures. *Ann. Surg.*, 97: 209, Feb. 1933.

SOUTTER, ROBERT: Reduction of Fractures of Long Bones. Apparatus for Obtaining General Relaxation of Soft Parts. *J. A. M. A.*, 94: 1547, May 17, 1935.

Chapter VIII

FRACTURES OF PELVIS. FRACTURES OF NECK OF FEMUR. DISLOCATIONS OF HIP. OTHER FRACTURES ABOUT HIP JOINT

FRACTURES of the pelvis are of importance because of static troubles and impairment of locomotion which follow immediately and as sequelae; because of injury to pelvic viscera which may be associated with the break and which may require immediate repair; and because

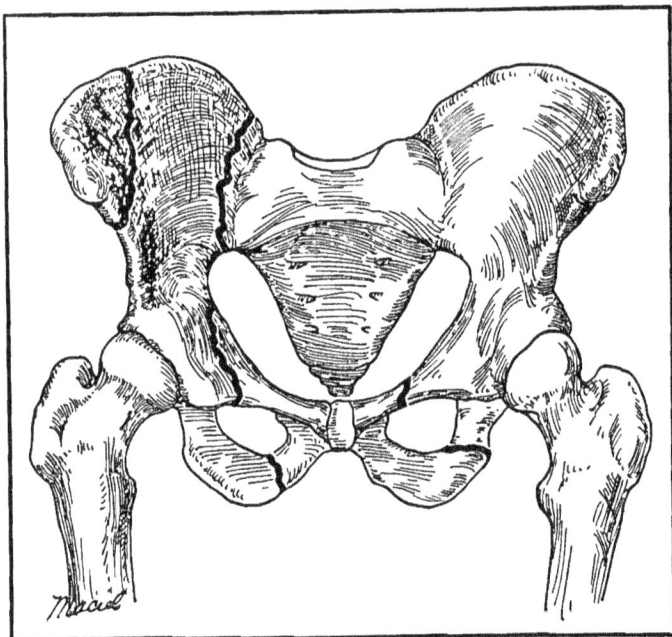

FIG. 41. Most common fractures of the pelvis.

of deformity of the pelvic outlet which may complicate parturition and delivery. They are brought about by crushing injuries, falls from a height, and localized trauma to a limited part of the pelvis.

The breaks may involve the wings of the ilium, the rhami of the pubis and the ischium, and, more rarely, the sacrum, and separation of the symphysis (Fig. 41).

74

Symptoms

The true nature and extent of a pelvic fracture can rarely be ascertained by examination, but require x-ray. The location of the fracture may often be approximated by the following tests:

1. Pressing the wings of the ilia together may elicit crepitus and mobility in the wings themselves and point tenderness in the pubic rhami and symphysis when fracture exists in those regions.

2. Pressure on the trochanters may disclose point tenderness in the hip joint, in the rhami of the pubes or ischii or symphysis.

3. Pressure over a separated pubic symphysis or fracture in that bone elicits point tenderness.

4. Pressure on the rhami of the pubes and tuberosities of the ischii causes pain in those regions when the fracture is in the rhami.

A pelvic injury of any extent is associated with considerable shock. Retroperitoneal hemorrhage of any considerable amount is often followed by intestinal paralysis and distension. A ruptured viscus may be suspected and is often extremely difficult to differentiate.

Complications

1. Rupture of the bladder.
2. Rupture of the urethra.
3. Paralytic ileus.
4. Rarely; damage to other pelvic viscera.

A proper examination after a pelvic injury should never omit inspection of a sample of urine (by catheter if none can be voided). If bloody urine is found, a catheter should be inserted and the bladder washed with salt solution. In this manner it can be determined if the bleeding comes from kidney, bladder or urethra. Failure to recover the salt solution injected indicates rupture of the bladder and this discovery should be followed by cystotomy, closure of the rent, and suprapubic drainage.

Ruptures of the urethra are disclosed by difficult catheterization. They should be repaired by perineal urethrotomy or the urethral channel may be re-established by combined urethral and retrograde catheterization; and an indwelling catheter may be left in position and the urethra allowed to heal around it.

Paralytic ileus is combated by stimulants, morphine, and such peristaltic excitants as pituitrin, pitressin, or eserine.

Treatment of the fracture will depend upon extent and location of the fracture. Breaks, which are not accompanied by separation of fragments, may be treated by rest in bed for six to eight weeks after which weight bearing is cautiously resumed.

Separation of the symphysis may sometimes be replaced by a tight swathe or sling in which the body is suspended (Fig. 42). The body weight causes lateral pressure which tends to compress the sides of the pelvis and push the pubic bones together. When the two pubic bones

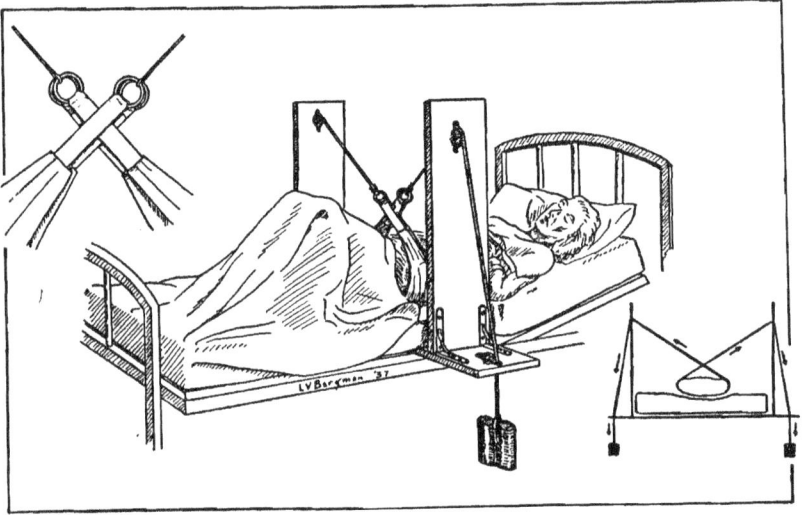

FIG. 42. A method of suspending and applying compression when necessary in treatment of fractures of the pelvis. Koster and Kassman. *J. Bone & Joint Surg.* 19-1130, Oct. 1937.

are displaced in both a lateral and atero-posterior direction, open fixation is often necessary.

When other bones of the pelvis are separated or displaced, reposition or improvement may be obtained by manipulation, using the legs as levers. A pin through the trochanter or through the wing of the ilium may be a useful way of attaching counter traction. After reposition has been attained, a cast from the axilla to the knees, with the thighs slightly flexed, is the most suitable fixation.

CENTRAL DISLOCATION OF THE HEAD OF THE FEMUR OR DEPRESSED FRACTURE OF THE ACETABULUM

This *uncommon injury* is due to falls on the trochanter. The author has seen four cases in which the victim was thrown forcibly against the side of an automobile when it struck an obstacle while skidding sideways. A positive diagnosis is not often possible except by x-ray. In two of our cases, it was made provisionally by noting the flattening of the trochanteric prominence on the affected side.

Reduction is made by traction on the leg in its long axis, while lateral traction is made by means of a swathe about the thigh. Counter traction is made by a sling about the perineum on which pull is made upward and outward. Position is best maintained by lateral traction with weights. These are attached by rope to a pin through the trochanter or a screw eye screwed into the trochanter. This device should be maintained for four weeks with bed rest continuing for two to four weeks.

This injury, while often followed by some pain in the hip and limb, is in many cases followed by restoration for comfortable use.

FRACTURE OF THE NECK OF THE FEMUR
INTRACAPSULAR FRACTURE OF THE
FEMUR (FIG. 43)

CAPITAL FRACTURE
INTERTROCHANTERIC FRACTURE OF THE
FEMUR (FIG. 44)

This fracture results from falls on the trochanter and, occasionally, by indirect violence. It occurs most commonly in the sixth decade, next on the seventh, then in the fifth, then in the eighth, and is one of the most distressing major catastrophies of the age. The true intracapsular fracture takes place between the head and the attachment of the neck

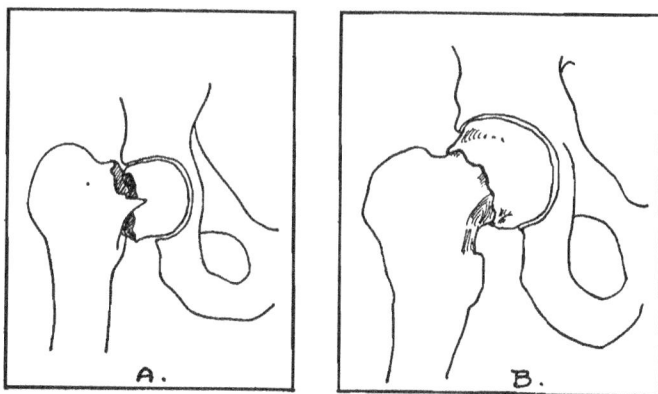

FIG. 43. Fracture of the neck of the femur. Intracapsular fracture. a) Displaced. b) Impacted.

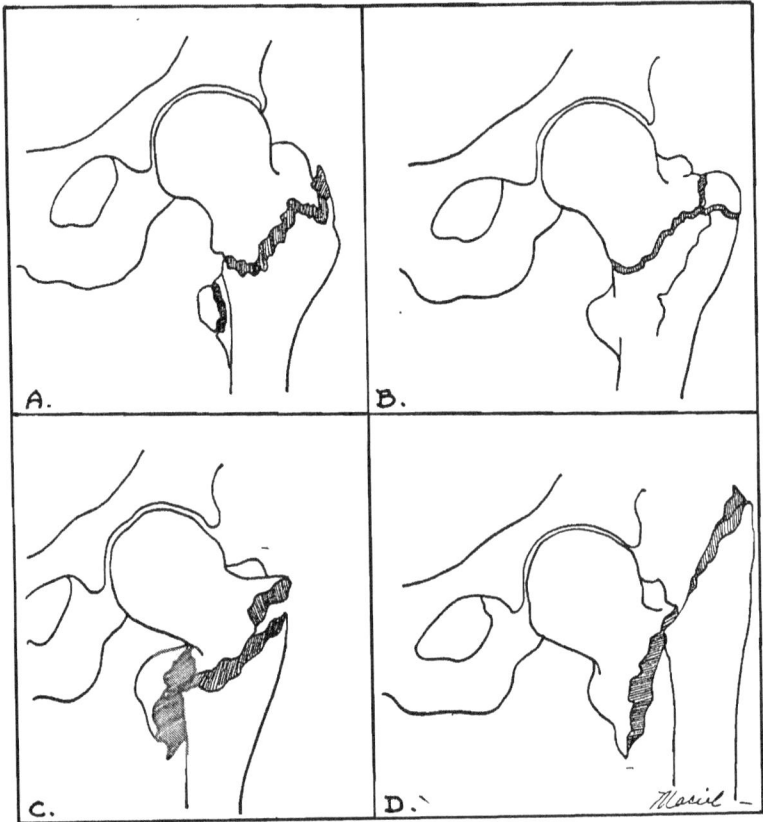

FIG. 44. Types of intertrochanteric fractures.

to the shaft. The intertrochanteric fracture is extracapsular but results from the same type of trauma, gives the same symptoms and is usually not distinguishable except by x-ray. The intracapsular fracture is frequently impacted.

SYMPTOMS AND SIGNS

After falling, the patient is unable to rise because of sharp pain in the hip. He lies with the foot everted and is unable to· turn the foot up (helpless eversion), nor is he able to raise the heel from the floor. On examining the hip, there is noted fullness in Scarpa's triangle, the adductors are tense, and the great trochanter is pulled upward and rotated backward. Measurement from the anterior superior spine to the internal malleolus shows the leg shorter than its fellow by from ¼″ to 1½″.

Fractures of the neck of the femur must be differentiated from:
1. Contusion of the hip.
2. Dislocation of the hip.
3. Fracture of the ischium or pubis.
4. Fracture of the acetabulum.
5. Fracture of the great trochanter.

The differentiation can usually be made if both hips and legs are exposed, compared, and measured carefully. Intracapsular fractures impacted in good position often cannot be positively differentiated without x-ray.

TREATMENT

Since these breaks often occur in patients enfeebled by advanced age, they will be unable to survive the rigor and confinement necessary to secure union. The most common fatal complication is hypostatic pneumonia.

When one of the following three conditions is present, rest in bed in the Fowler position is the proper treatment.

1. When the fracture is impacted in good position, i.e., not more than ¾″ shortening and slight eversion.

2. When the patient is very feeble and prolonged recumbency would be apt to cause a fatal termination by hypostatic pneumonia.

3. When the patient is obese or does not have control of sphincters.

It is customary when treatment by bed rest only is carried out to immobilize the leg with sand bags. These we feel are little more than a placebo and are uncomfortable and may as well be omitted. We prefer instead the *anti-eversion boot* (Fig. 48).

When the patient's general condition will permit it, *the Whitman abduction treatment* in a plaster spica is the one which has given the greatest (Figs. 46 & 47) number of good results. Under the general or spinal anesthesia the fracture is reduced by the *manipulation of Leadbetter* (Fig. 45). The thigh is flexed to a right angle and traction is made upward. The thigh is rotated inward by turning the flexed leg outward. The thigh and knee are straightened and traction is made in the long axis of the femur, abducted to the limit.

If reduction has been satisfactory, the foot will not turn outward when the heel rests unsupported laterally in the palm of the hand. A plaster spica is applied to the body and the abducted leg from the axilla to the foot, with the foot well inverted and the knees slightly flexed (Figs. 46 & 47).

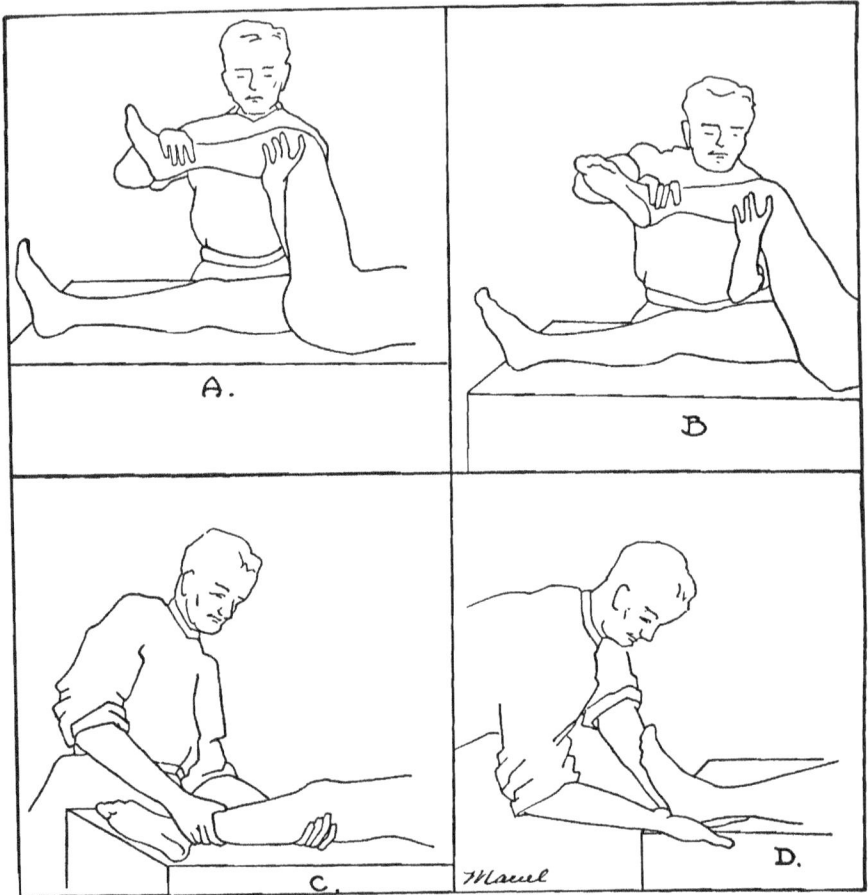

FIG. 45. Leadbetter's maneuvers for reduction of fracture of the femur. a) Thigh is flexed to a right angle to the body and the knee to the same angle and traction is made upward. b) While pulling upward the thigh is rotated inward, using the leg as a lever. c) Leg and thigh are straightened in wide abduction. d) When fragments are accurately reduced and thigh is abducted the foot will remain upright on the palm of the hand without support.

In this position the femur is stabilized by the great trochanter pressing on the rim of the acetabulum and the tense adductors, acting as a fulcrum, cause the broken surfaces to be pressed together when the thigh is abducted.

This cast should be worn eight weeks and after removal the patient should spend four weeks in bed. He may then be in a chair for four weeks and can then use crutches. *No weight bearing should be permitted until six months.*

In the past few years several procedures have been introduced for pinning the fragments of the hip fracture together without exposing the fracture. The steps are as follows:

Twenty to forty c.c. of 2 per cent procaine are injected into the capsule

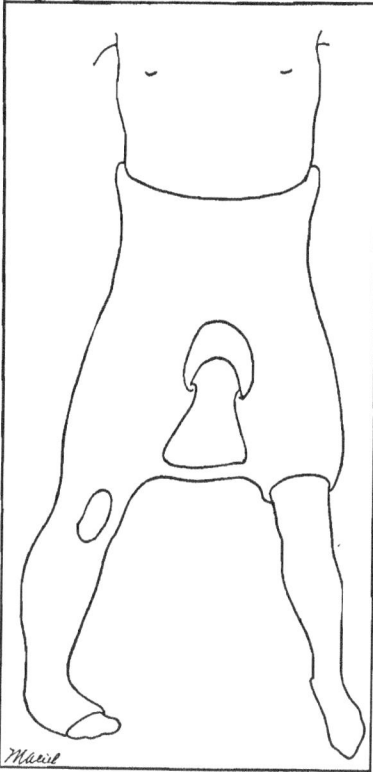

FIG. 46. Whitman abduction spica cast. Double. Note inversion of leg. When cast includes good leg and cross bar is used, the cast need not extend above the brim of the pelvis.

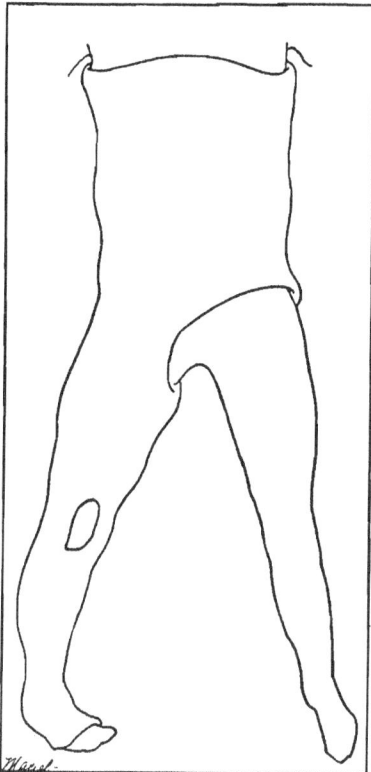

FIG. 47. Whitman abduction spica cast. Single. When good leg is not included, cast must extend to axilla to maintain abduction.

of the hip joint after which the part will be sufficiently painless to permit a reduction after the method of Leadbetter. This reduction is checked, however, by portable x-ray on the operating table. An incision is then made over the trochanter and about four inches long. The soft tissues over the bone are separated and the pins or screws for fixation are then inserted by rotation or driving. They extend through the trochanter and neck into the head. The position of the pins or screws is then checked by x-ray and the wound is closed. No cast or other external fixation is applied. The patient is allowed upon crutches as soon as the wound has healed.

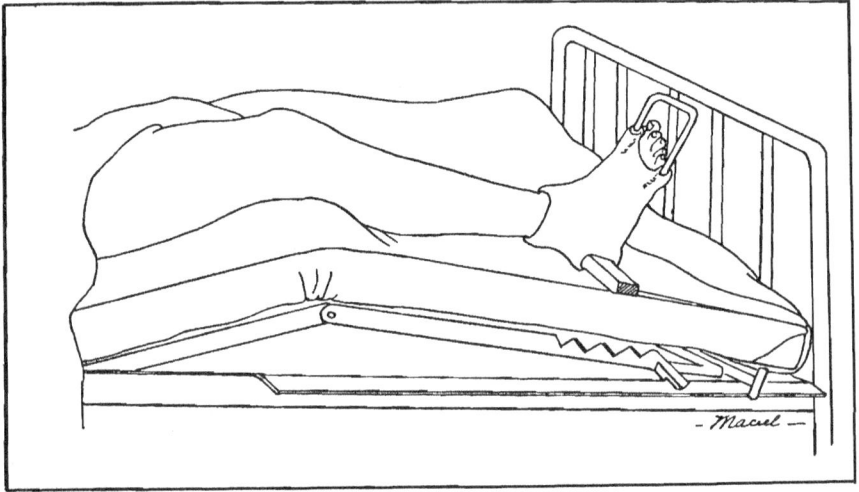

FIG. 48. Anti-eversion boot. Illustration of the anti-eversion boot which is used instead of sand bags in the treatment of impacted fractures of the neck of the femur when a plaster case is inadvisable. A well-padded boot of plaster is applied and a cross bar of wood is incorporated so that the foot cannot rotate. The loop of wire extending above the toes keeps the bed clothes off the toes and obviates the troublesome bed cradle. This loop is put in all leg cases when the patient is confined to bed. Author's article on Treatment of Fractures in Cincinnati General Hospital. *Ann. Surg.* 97:2-164, Feb. 1933.

The most frequently used pins are:

1. The single three flanged pin of Smith Peterson (Fig. 50).
2. The three or four steel pins of Austin Moore (Fig. 49).
3. One or two long slender wood screws (Fig. 51).

This method of fixation promises to be a great advance in the management of these cases for the reason that it is a comparatively minor surgical procedure. The patient is allowed up on crutches in a few days and can get about on crutches or a wheel chair and no atrophy of the leg muscles or fixation of the knee joint follows as is the case when prolonged fixation in a cast is employed.

A sufficient number of cases have been observed to determine that this method is followed by a higher proportion of union in the intracapsular fractures than by other methods of treatment.

While intracapsular fractures and intertrochanteric fractures are similar types of deformity and symptoms and require the same treatment,
they differ strongly in prognosis.

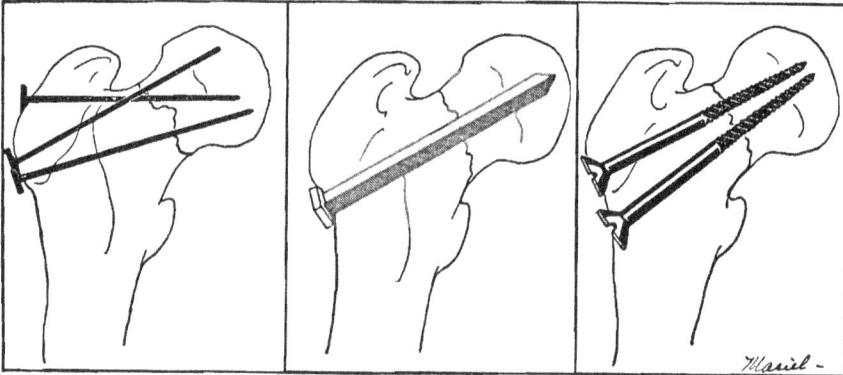

FIGS. 49, 50, 51. Three common methods for open fixation of fracture of neck of femur.
49.) Austin Moore pins. 50.) Smith-Peterson nail. 51.) Wood screws.

Intertrochanteric fractures nearly always unite and are followed by
good functional results *if a good reduction has been secured.* Intracapsular fractures are followed by a high proportion of failure of union
even where a perfect reduction has been made and the treatment has

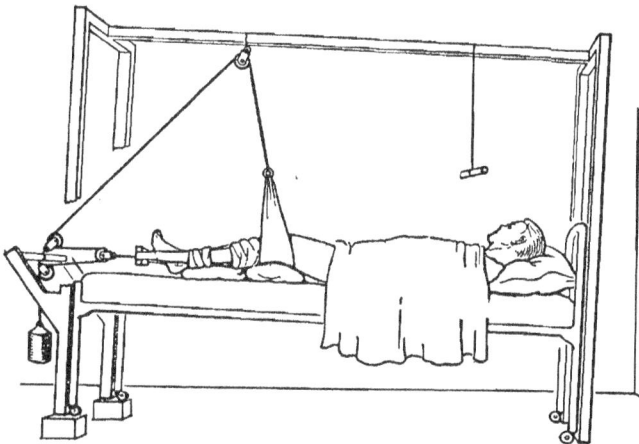

FIG. 52. Russell traction.

been adequate. The reason for this is that in some cases the fracture tears or occludes the nutrient artery to the head and neck which enters the bone on the posterior surface at the junction of the head and neck. When this happens, if the small artery which enters the head of the femur through the ligamentum teres is inadequate, aseptic necrosis of the head and neck follow and these structures are absorbed.

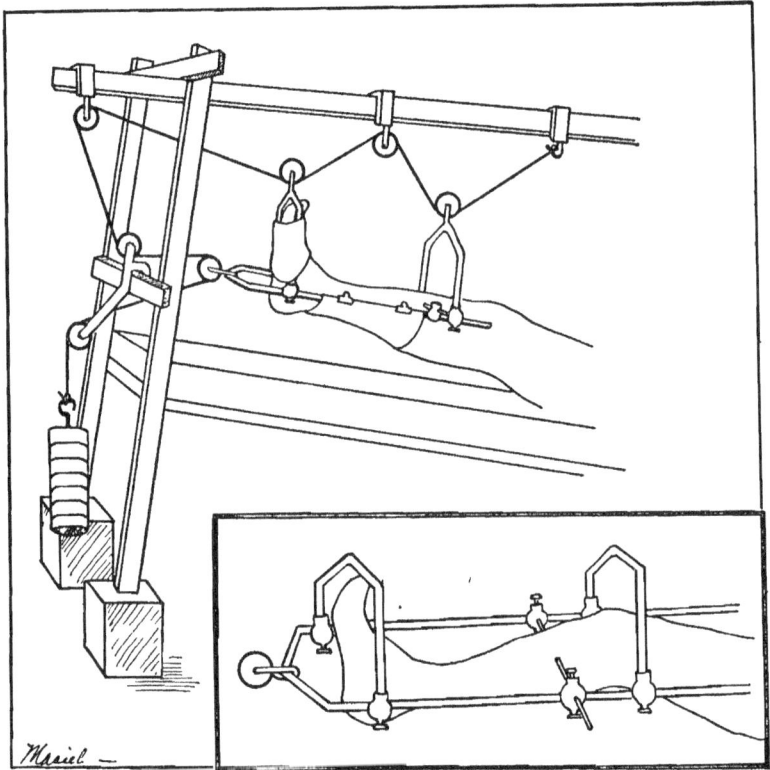

FIG. 53. Author's modification of Russell traction. Leg cannot rotate and there is no sling about the popliteal space imperiling circulation of the foot and leg.

Intertrochanteric fractures may also be treated by some form of balanced traction. Our preference is for the method of Russell (Fig. 52), or the Russell principle which we have modified so as to use skeletal traction (Fig. 53). Obviously such treatment can only be carried out in a patient who can stand confinement in bed for six weeks or more.

DISLOCATION OF THE HIP JOINT

This is an uncommon accident constituting but two per cent of all dislocations. There are two major varieties, anterior and posterior. In each of these the head may lie in one of two positions:

Anterior   Low or thyroid foramen
                High or pubic
Posterior   Low or sciatic notch
                High or dorsum of ilium

The posterior dislocation is much more frequent than the anterior. The anterior dislocation results from violent hyperabduction of the hip. The thigh and knee are flexed and the leg is rotated outwardly. In the high position the head may be felt on the pubis. The prominence of the trochanter is missing and the hip appears flattened.

Reduction: Several methods may be used. All depend on relaxing the capsule and causing the head to traverse its course in reverse direction. Deep anesthesia should be employed. All methods begin with flexion of the thigh and leg. First abduct slightly and pull the thigh at a right angle to the body, rotate the thigh inward, abduct the thigh, and extend the entire leg.

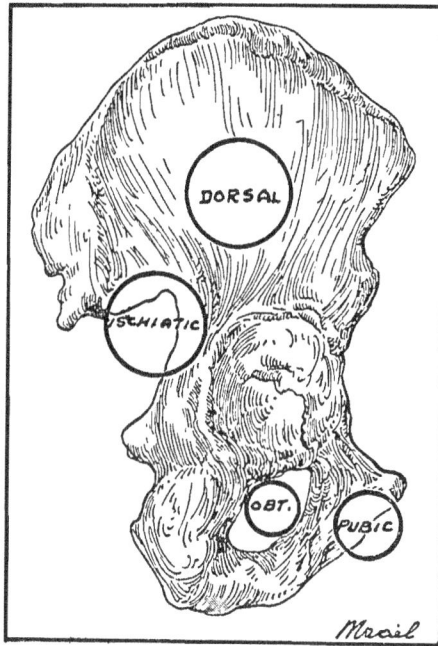

FIG. 54. Diagram showing dislocations of the head of the femur.

Posterior dislocation: This displacement occurs when force is applied to the leg when the thigh is flexed adducted and rotated internally. Typical accidents are mine and excavation cave-ins when the patient is stooping and a mass falls on his back, and automobile collisions when the patient is thrown forward and his knee strikes the back of the front seat or the instrument board. The knee and thigh are slightly flexed and the leg is rotated internally. The great toe will often rest naturally on the instep of the opposite foot and the leg will be shortened.

REDUCTION

Deep relaxing anesthesia should be administered. The knee and thigh should be flexed to 90°. Adduct the thigh and rotate internally. Lift one thigh upward and rotate outward.

After treatment: Rest in bed for six weeks is all that is required, though abduction of the leg should be prevented by sand bag or binding the legs together. Complete activity should not be resumed for six to eight weeks.

Fracture of the great trochanter occurs by direct violence and occasionally by avulsion. It is frequently impacted and, when not, the loosened fragment is drawn upward by the glutei.

Diagnosis is made by point tenderness and exclusion of other possibilities such as fracture of the neck of the femur and dislocation. An x-ray is necessary to be certain.

TREATMENT

When impacted, rest in bed is all that is required. When detached, the thigh should be splinted in flexion and eversion. Open fixation gives the most satisfactory replacement and the shortest convalescence.

Fracture of the lesser trochanter is by avulsion. Diagnosis cannot certainly be made without x-ray. Treatment is rest in bed with the thigh sharply flexed for three to four weeks.

REFERENCES

CALDWELL, JOHN A.: Fracture of the Neck of the Femur. Treatment by Immediate Fixation. *Ohio State M. J.,* 33: 30-34, Jan. 1937.

CHANDLER, S. B. and KREUSCHER, P. H.: A Study of the Blood Supply of the Ligamentum Teres and Its Relation to the Circulation of the Head of the Femur. *J. Bone & Joint Surg.,* 14: 834, 1932.

COTTON, F. J.: Intracapsular Hip Fracture. *Bone & Joint Surg.,* 16: 105, Jan. 1934.

CUBBINS, W. R., CONLEY, A. H., CALLAHAN, J. J.: Fractures of the Acetabulum. *Surg., Gynec. & Obst.,* 15: 387, Sept. 1930.

KOSTER, HARRY, and KASMAN, LOUIS P.: Treatment of Fractures of the Pelvis. *J. Bone & Joint Surg.,* 19, 4: 1130, Oct. 1937.

LEADBETTER, G. W.: A Treatment of Fractures of the Neck of the Femur. *J. Bone & Joint Surg.,* 15: 931, Oct. 1933.

MOORE, AUSTIN T.: Fracture of the Hip Joint (Intracapsular). New Method of Treatment. *Internat. S. Digest,* 19: 323-330, June 1935.

NOLAND, LLOYD, and CONWELL, H. E.: Fractures of the Pelvis. *Surg., Gynec. & Obst.,* 56: 522, Feb. 15, 1933.

PHEMISTER, D. B.: Fractures of the Neck of the Femur. *Surg., Gynec. & Obst.,* 59: 415, 1934.

SEVER, J. W.: Traumatic Separation of the Symphysis Pubis. *New England J. Med.,* 204: 355, Feb. 19, 1931.

SMITH, PETERSEN N. M., CAVE, E. F. and VAN GORDER, G. W.: Treatment by Internal Fixation. *Arch. Surg.,* 23: 715, Nov. 1931.

WHITMAN, ROYAL: Abduction Treatment of Fracture of Neck of Femur. *Surg., Gynec. & Obst.,* 27: 578, Dec. 1918.

WHITMAN, ROYAL: Fractures of the Neck of the Femur. *Ann. Surg.,* 53: 489, 1911.

WOLCOTT, W. E.: Circulation of the Head and Neck of the Femur. *J. A. M. A.,* 100: 27, Jan. 7, 1933.

Chapter IX

FRACTURES OF SHAFT OF FEMUR IN ADULTS AND CHILDREN. SEPARATION OF LOWER FEMORAL EPIPHYSIS. FRACTURES OF FEMORAL CONDYLES. FRACTURES AND DISLOCATIONS OF PATELLA

FRACTURES of the shaft of the femur result from direct violence, from muscular action, and are a frequent gunshot fracture. The location of the break is usually designated as follows:

1. Sub-trochanteric.
2. Upper third.
3. Middle third.
4. Lower third.
5. Supracondylar.
6. Condylar.

In fractures above the upper third, the psoas and illiacus muscles flex and evert the upper fragment. In breaks about the middle or higher, the adductors draw the upper fragment inward.

In those fractures close to the knee, the calf muscles draw the lower fragment back into the popliteal space.

SYMPTOMS

All symptoms of fracture are present, and since the femur is a large bone buried in large muscles, fracture is often associated with great swelling, ecchymosis, and severe shock.

TREATMENT

Preliminary: No fracture of the femur should be moved or handled without some fixation of the leg. *By far the most effective emergency splint is the Thomas knee splint* (Fig. 55). The general adoption of this splint in the British Army and its application on the battle field before moving the patient reduced the mortality in gunshot fractures of the femur from 80 per cent to 20 per cent. When this splint is not available, *a long Liston splint* accomplishes some fixation. This is a board reaching from the axilla to the foot, and the leg and body are bandaged to it. If nothing else can be done, some restriction of motion can be effected

88

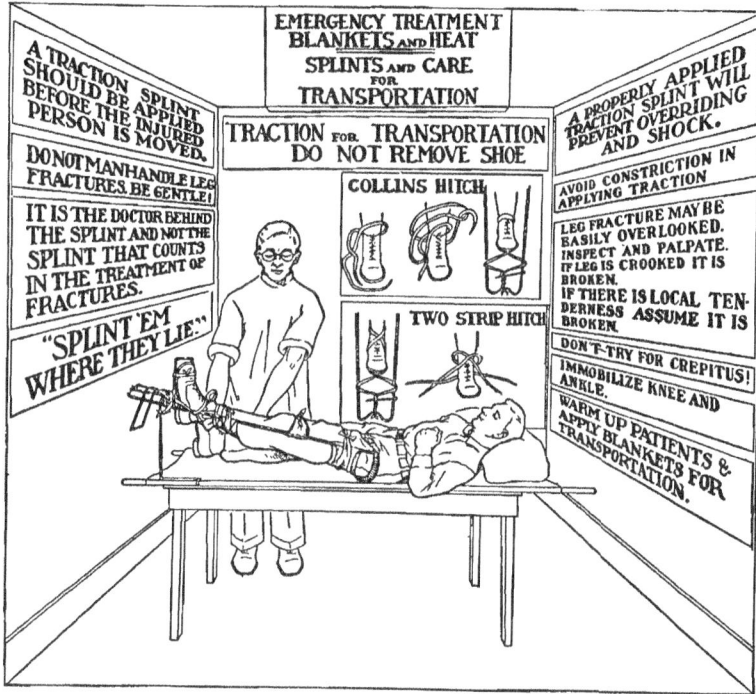

FRACTURE OF THE LOWER EXTREMITY: EMERGENCY TREATMENT

Early splintage and application of traction will lessen deformity, decrease shock, and make early and complete reduction of fragments easy to accomplish. The fault today in emergency treatment is not that it is not well done but that it is not applied soon enough. The injured person is picked up and transported to home or hospital without regard to the fracture. It is a common experience to see a person with a fracture of the femoral shaft arrive at the admission ward of a hospital with from 2 to 4 inches of overriding of fragments. This is proved to be unnecessary by the few patients who arrive in a Thomas splint. Some intelligent physician applied the Thomas splint before the patient was picked up, with the result that there was practically no pain, no overriding of fragments, and less shock. There was ample evidence of the advantage of early splintage and traction gained on the fields of France in the great war.

FIG. 55. Fractures of the lower extremity. Emergency treatment. From *Primer on Fractures*. Cooperative Committee on Fractures. American Medical Association.

by tightly lashing both legs together. Any splint which reaches only to the perineum is of very little effect since it does not restrict rotation.

Practically all fractures of the femur can be treated by one of the following methods:

1. Immediate reduction and immobilization by cast. *This must always be a spica and include the foot to prevent rotation.* While this method

is ideal, when possible, it can only be carried out when the fragments
are near enough transverse to remain engaged. To carry out this treatment requires equipment for putting on a spica cast, skill in handling
plaster, and easily accessible x-ray facilities for checking the reduction.

2. The fracture may be reduced and held in a Thomas splint by
slings and fixed traction and a cast may be applied later. However, the
padded ring on a Thomas splint is uncomfortable and makes nursing
difficult. *It is entirely inapplicable in women.* When reduction is not

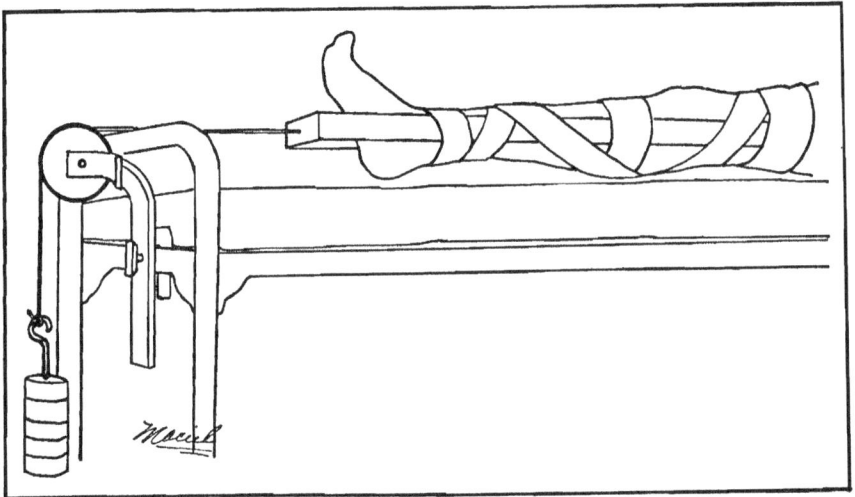

FIG. 56. Buck's extension. Counter traction made by elevating the foot of the bed.

possible, some form of traction is necessary. The oldest and most used
method is by the *Buck's extension* (Fig. 56), in which the leg lies in
bed, adhesive plaster is applied to the skin and traction on this is
made by means of weights hanging on a cord which passes over a pulley
attached to the foot of the bed. From 20 to 40 pounds are necessary,
depending on the muscular development of the patient and the nature
of the break.

Buck's extension is objectionable for the following reasons: The leg
must lie straight, which is not the position of rest and muscular relaxation and, furthermore, traction can be made in only one plane—that of
the bed and, since the leg is fastened to the bed, movement of the
patient in bed moves the fragments on each other.

Balanced traction—in which the limb is suspended and counter balanced and traction is made in the long axis of the femur. There are many devices and systems for suspension for balanced traction. A few in most common use will be mentioned:

1. Thomas splint with the Pearson attachment for flexing the knee (Fig. 57).
2. Hodgkin's suspension splint.
3. Russell traction (Figs. 52 & 53).

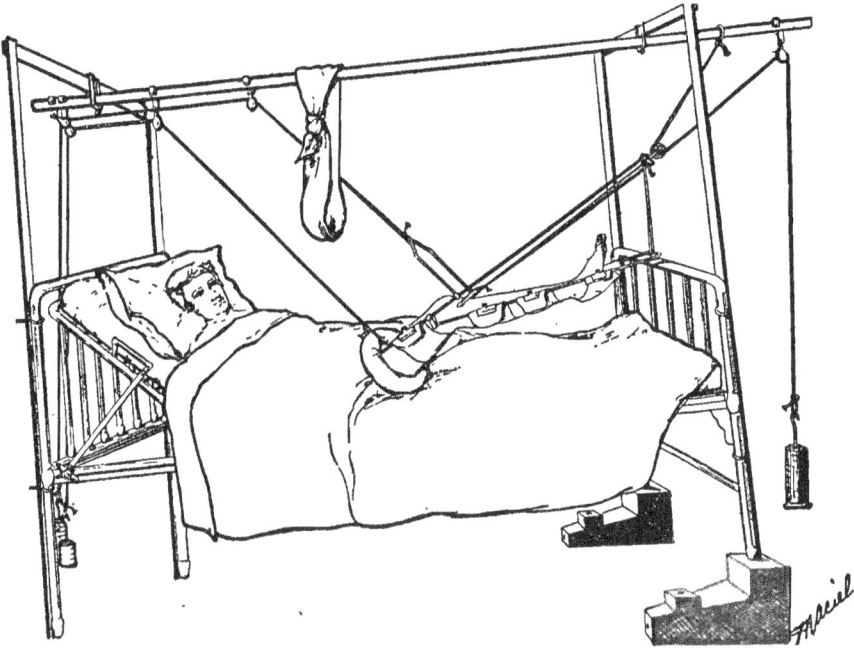

FIG. 57. A method of balanced traction under the Balkan frame. Illustration of the usual method of treating fractures of the shaft of the femur—a Thomas splint with the Pearson attachment. The Steinman pin is inserted through the head of the tibia, but when there is special reason it is occasionally passed through the lower end of the femur.

Traction may be made by adhesive plaster to the skin or skeletal traction by means of Steinman pin, Kirschner wire or ice tongs. Our preference is for Steinman pin, *which should always be bored in, never driven*. Whichever is used may be inserted into the condyles of the femur, the tibia at the level of the tubercle or the os calcis. Skeletal traction is much more effective than skin traction and far more comfortable.

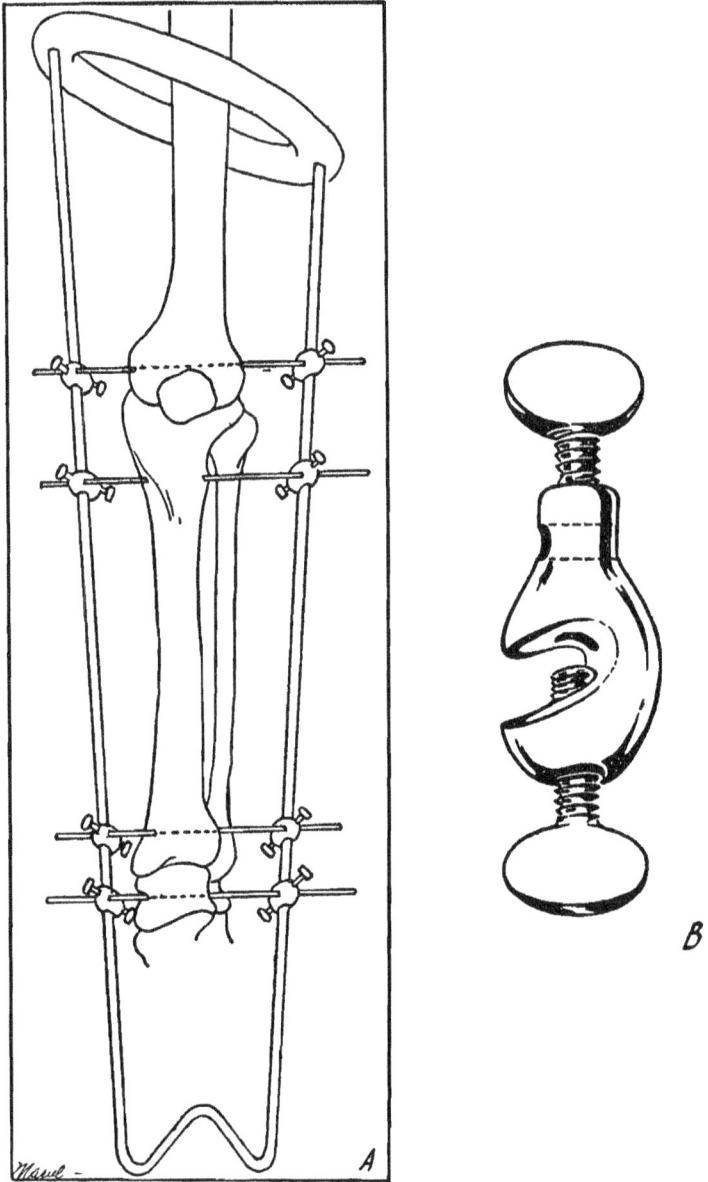

FIG. 58. Drawing showing method of fixation and traction by using Steinman pin fastened to sides of Thomas splint with author's pin lugs. a) Pin through condyles of femur. b) Through tibia at level of tubercle. c) Through tibia at ankle. d) Through os calcis.

When instituting traction on a fractured femur (or any other bone), the maximum weight should be applied at once and then diminished when the purpose is accomplished. When muscles once contract and become infiltrated with blood, much more pull is required to overcome the muscle effort.

Traction should be maintained three to six weeks and then may be replaced by a cast or walking calliper (Fig. 59). A patient with a fractured femur should not bear weight earlier than twelve weeks and then only when the union is firm and the x-ray shows dense callus, adequate in amount.

Occasionally, fractures of the femur can be satisfactorily put together *only by open operation.* Sub-trochanteric fractures and supra-condylar breaks are most likely to require this treatment. When open operation is necessary, it should only be done by one with experience, working with good facilities and complete instruments.

FRACTURES OF THE FEMUR IN CHILDREN

In children and adolescents, the period before completion of bone growth, callus forms rapidly and any excess is absorbed readily so that what appears in an x-ray of a recent fracture as gross misalignment will eventually result in firm union and no deformity in a break of a single bone such as the femur. Some shortening, often as much as one inch, will be followed by an increased growth of bone so that the shortened leg will often be longer than its fellow in the course of a year or two. For these reasons a failure to secure accurate reduction should not occasion the same apprehension that a similar result would in an adult. Open fixation is rarely necessary, particularly

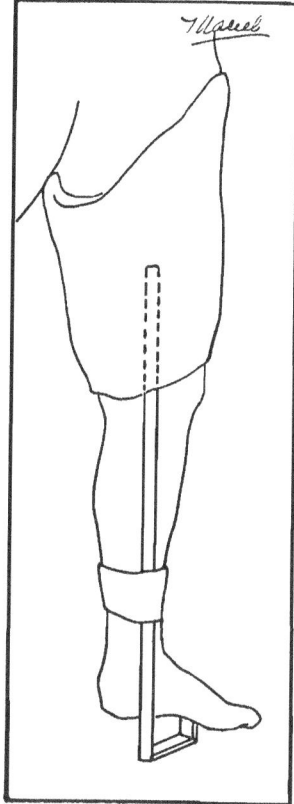

FIG. 59. Walking calliper. A plaster cuff well padded to bear weight on the tuberosity of the ischium is applied from knee to perineum. An iron bar $\frac{1}{8}''$ x $\frac{1}{2}''$ is incorporated in the cuff and extends one inch below the heel. A cork sole $\frac{3}{4}''$ thick is put on the shoe for the good leg.

since children do not tolerate well the shock occasioned by extensive bone operations.

Children up to eight or nine years are best treated for femoral fractures by *Bryant suspension* (Fig. 60). In this the thigh is suspended at an angle of 90° to the body and held there by counterweight. The weight of the body makes counter traction. This treatment is suitable so

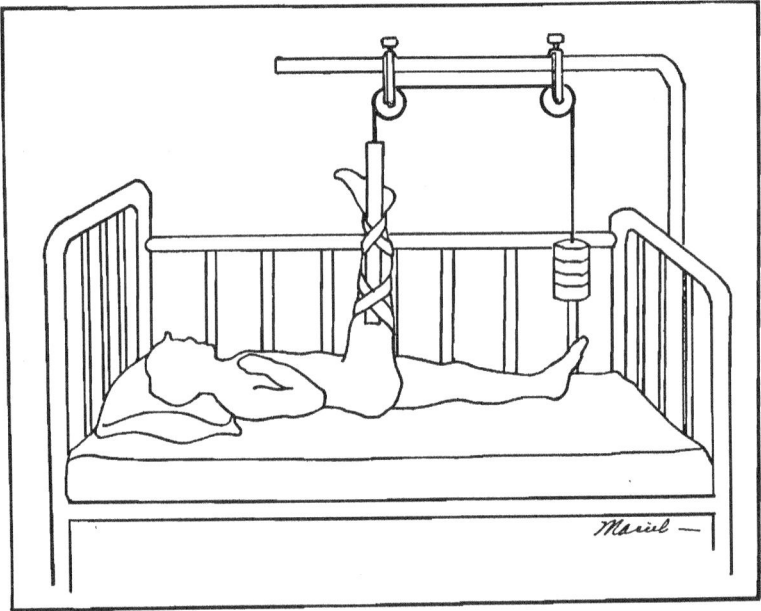

FIG. 60. Bryant suspension method of treatment of fracture of the femur in children.

long as the thigh can be flexed to a right angle without flexing the knee. Ability to do this usually passes at about 8 or 9 years. In a doubtful case the uninjured thigh should be flexed to 90° and, if the knee can be kept straight when the thigh is so flexed, the case is suitable for Bryant suspension (Fig. 61). Treatment is quite comfortable for the patient and nursing is facilitated. It should be continued for four to six weeks, then a cast should be applied. In very restless children, both legs should be suspended. When the thigh cannot be flexed to 90° without flexing the knee, some other method may be used. This may be another form of traction or reduction and a cast. In older children, the same methods should be followed as in adults.

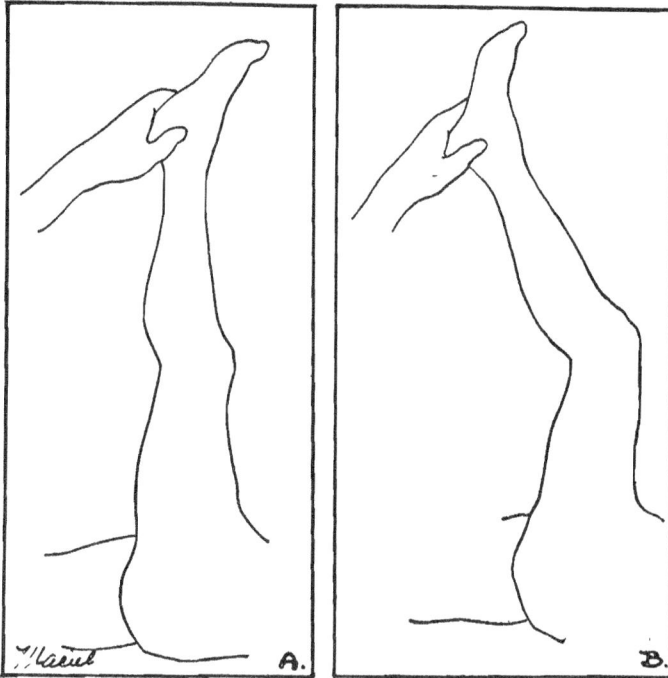

FIG. 61. Test maneuver to determine applicability of Bryant suspension method. a) With thigh flexed to right angle, knee can be fully extended. Bryant method is applicable. b) With thigh flexed to right angle, knee cannot be fully extended. The Bryant method can rarely be used in children more than seven years old.

Fractures of the femur in infants are best treated in a *Van Arsdale cast* (Fig. 63).

FRACTURE OF THE LOWER EPIPHYSIS

This accident occurs before the 18th year and is due to extreme direct violence. The epiphysis is nearly always displaced onto the anterior surface of the femur. Reduction is accomplished by traction in hyperextension and then flexion, while traction is continued (Fig. 63b). After reduction, the knee is flexed on

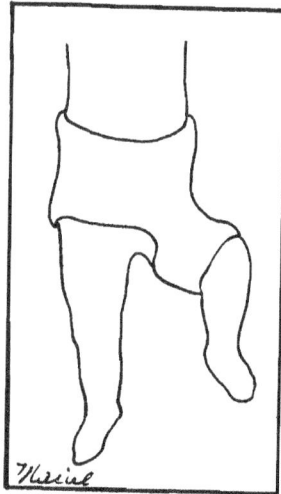

FIG. 62. Van Arsdale cast. Dressing for fracture of a femur in an infant.

the thigh and held by a cast or bandage. When reduction cannot be made, open replacement should not be delayed. There is danger that the popliteal artery, which is stretched over the ragged edge of the upper fragment, will be eroded if the deformity is allowed to persist (Fig. 63 a).

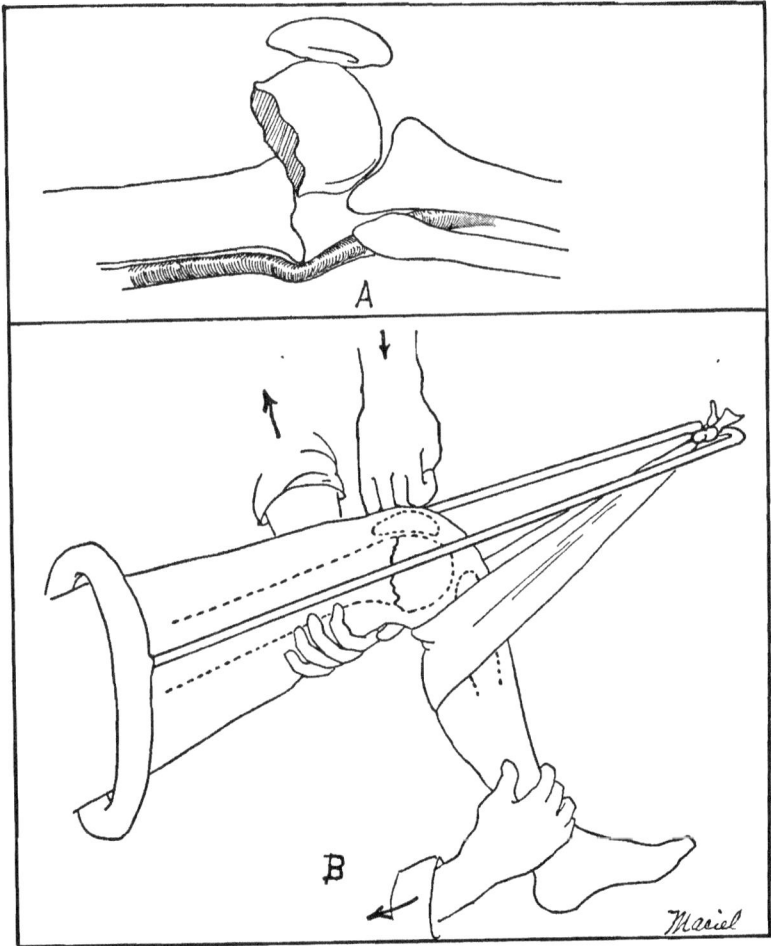

FIG. 63. Separation of lower epiphysis of femur. a) Showing usual anterior displacement and how this may be followed by erosion of the popliteal artery. b) Showing method of reducing anterior displacement of lower epiphysis.

FRACTURES OF THE CONDYLES OF THE FEMUR

One or both condyles may be broken. Symptoms: Owing to the close proximity to the joint and the distension of the knee by bloody effusion, *diagnosis is rarely possible except by x-ray* (Fig. 64).

When there is great displacement, traction with the leg straight in a Thomas splint or Buck's extension will often bring about reposition. When this is not successful, open fixation is called for. The knee should

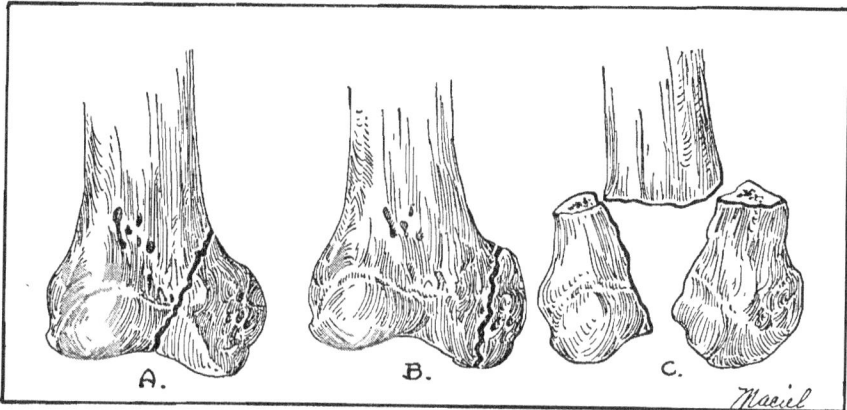

FIG. 64. Types of fracture of condyles of the femur.

be immobilized for at least six weeks in a cast. Effusion into the knee joint should be reduced by aspiration.

FRACTURE OF THE PATELLA

This fracture is brought about in two ways:

1. By muscular action. Sudden contraction of the quadriceps tendon, as in trying to regain balance after slipping, pulls the patella in two, in a more or less transverse direction and the lateral expansions of the quadriceps tendon are usually torn. Occasionally, instead of the patella being fractured, the patellar tendon is torn and, more rarely, the quadriceps tendon will be pulled off the patella.

2. By direct trauma. Falls or blows on the patella when the quadriceps tendon is tense. Automobile collisions in which the driver or front seat passenger is thrown forcibly forward, striking his kneecap on the edge of the instrument board, is often a method of patellar fracture today.

SYMPTOMS

The knee is swollen from effusion into the joint. A groove may be felt in the surface of the patella if the fragments are separated and the groove may be widened when the knee is flexed, or when the patient attempts to extend the knee. Power of extension is lost only when the lateral expansions of the quadriceps tendon are torn.

TREATMENT

When an x-ray taken with the knee flexed shows the patellar fragments separated or when the separation between fragments can be felt, and when ability to extend the knee is lost, open fixation should be done without delay. The patella is exposed, best we think by a transverse incision, the fragments are firmly united by wire, heavy catgut, silk or kangaroo tendon, or autogenous suture material. The tears in the quadriceps tendon are repaired and a Schantz dressing is applied. The patient can walk in ten to fourteen days *but should be cautioned not to flex the knee.* Fixation in extension, we think, is not necessary and delays restoration of function after the fixation is removed.

When the patellar fracture is not separated and power of extension persists, a Schantz dressing with ten to fourteen days rest of the joint is sufficient treatment, *except that flexion of the knee should be forbidden.* When operation is not done at once, or is not necessary at all, distension of the knee joint should be relieved by aspiration as should distension of this joint from any other cause.

We feel very strongly that strapping or bandaging a fracture of the patella to approximate fragments should not be done because it is ineffectual and may cause skin irritation which would delay operation. In most fractures of the patella, shreds of the capsule fall into the chasm between the fragments and so prevent their approximation and body union.

DISLOCATION OF THE PATELLA

This occurs in childhood and *usually to the outer side.* Dislocation to the inner side is rare. It is apt to recur and become habitual. The deformity is evident.

Reduction is made by flexing the thigh and extending the knee to relax the quadriceps tendon when the patella may be manipulated into position. Habitual dislocation of the patella requires plastic repair of the patellar tendon.

REFERENCES

ANDRUS, WILLIAM D.: Fractures of the Shaft of the Femur. *Ann. Surg.* 80: 848, Dec. 1924.

BROOKE, R.: The Treatment of Fracture of the Patella by Excision. *Brit. J. Surg.*, 96: 733, Apr. 1937.

CALDWELL, JOHN A.: Fractures of the Femur in Children. *J. Med.*, Cincinnati, Ohio, Jan. 1935.

CONWELL, H. E.: Acute Fractures Shaft of Femur in Children. *J. Bone & Joint Surg.*, 11: 593, Jan. 1929.

GALLIE, W. E.: The Late Repair of Fractures of the Patella & Rupture of the Ligamentum Patellae and Quadriceps Tendon. *J. Bone & Joint Surg.*, 9: 47, Jan. 1927.

JOHNSTON, L. B.: The Treatment of Fractures of the Femur in Children. *Arch. Surg.*, 10: 730, March 1925.

PEARSON and DRUMMOND: *Fractured Femurs, Their Treatment by Calliper Extension.* London, 1919.

RUSSELL, R. H.: Fracture of the Femur. *Brit. J. Surg.*, 11: 491, Jan. 1924.

Chapter X

FRACTURES OF TIBIA AND FIBULA. POTT'S FRACTURE
AND OTHER FRACTURES ABOUT ANKLE JOINT.
DISLOCATION OF ANKLE. FRACTURES OF
ASTRAGALUS. OS CALCIS. TARSAL BONES.
METATARSALS AND PHALANGES

A T THE upper end, either the external or internal condyles of the tibia
may be broken. When the external condyle is broken, the head of
the fibula is usually either cracked or broken off. The shaft of either or
both bones may be broken at any point.

There are two classical types of fractures of the tibia and fibula: (1)
Spiral or Torsion fracture; (2) Pott's fracture.

FRACTURE OF THE CONDYLES (FIG. 65)

These may occur by avulsion from forcible lateral bending of the knee
joint or may occur from direct violence. In the latter case, the fragments

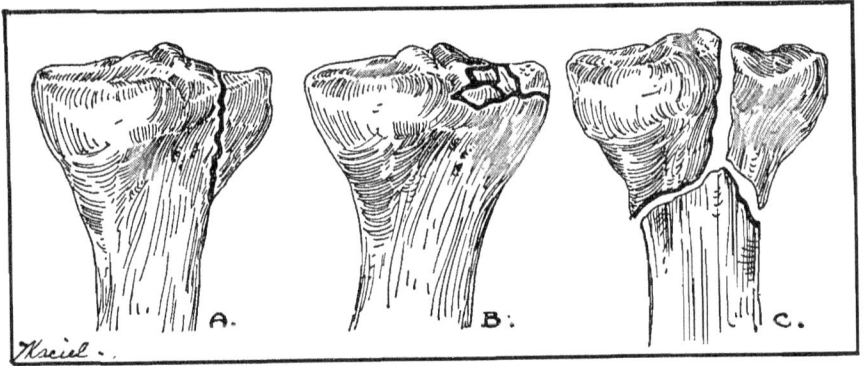

Fig. 65. Types of fractures of head of the tibia involving the articular surface.

are often comminuted. A common combined cause is the bumper fracture
in which an automobile bumper strikes the head of the fibula and com-
minutes it together with the outer condyle of the tibia, while the inner
condyle is torn off by the forcible stretching of the internal lateral ligament when the knee is bent laterally.

SYMPTOMS

There is great effusion into the knee joint. Point tenderness is felt over one or both tibial condyles. Lateral motion of the knee joint is increased. Mobility and crepitus of the fragments may sometimes be felt.

TREATMENT

A Schanz dressing with sharp elevation of the leg is *an excellent early treatment*. This dressing immobilizes the knee joint, compresses the fragments together, and keeps down effusion. After a day or two, the knee joint should be aspirated if there is much effusion, and the dressing may be reapplied and aspiration repeated if there seems much likelihood of the effusion recurring.

The best permanent dressing is a cast from perineum to toes with the knee slightly flexed. If the fragments are much separated, attempt may be made to replace them by clamping. If this is not successful, open operation should be done and the displaced fragment put into position and fixed by wire, nail or bone peg, or bolt through the condyles.

The cast should be worn for six weeks. Weight bearing should not begin for four weeks or more. After removal of the cast, gentle active movements should be begun to restore motion in the knee.

COMPLICATIONS AND SEQUELAE

1. The peroneal nerve is sometimes injured as it winds around the head of the fibula. This is shown by foot drop and numbness on the outer side and dorsum of the foot. This injury may result from the original trauma or from pressure by a tight cast or splint.

2. Ankylosis or restricted motion in the knee joint.

3. Instability of the knee joint with increased lateral motion.

4. Absorption of one condyle which is followed by genu valgus or varum, depending on which condyle is involved.

Treatment of complications: Peroneal nerve injury should be followed by exploration of the nerve if signs of improvement are not shown in four or six weeks. The other complications are usually caused by insufficient immobilization and too early weight bearing.

FRACTURES OF THE SHAFT OF THE TIBIA AND FIBULA

These may be located in any part of the bone; are often comminuted; or open fractures and section fractures are frequently encountered.

SYMPTOMS

All symptoms are readily elicited except possibly when the break is of the green-stick or subperiosteal variety, or when the fibula or tibia alone is broken. In the latter case the unbroken bone will splint the fracture and reduce the mobility in the break. Diagnosis may then depend on point tenderness and x-ray.

TREATMENT

When the fracture is nearly or completely transverse, it should be reduced by manipulation and a cast or Stimson splint should be applied

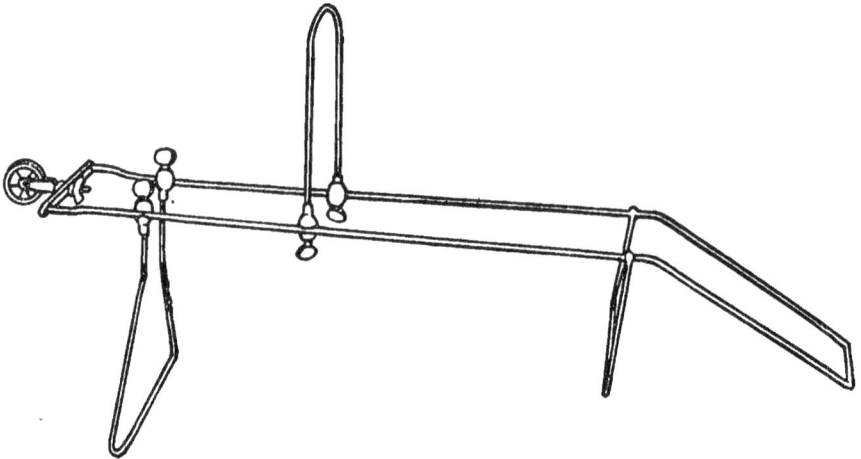

FIG. 66. Author's knee flexion splint. A simple device which serves the purpose of the more cumbersome and expensive Braun Frame. By attaching another "croquet wicket" the entire device may be suspended. Treatment of Fractures in Cincinnati General Hospital. *Ann. Surg.* 97-2-161-176, Feb. 1933.

from perineum to foot. The knee should be flexed to 135°. When reduction is impossible owing to obliquity or comminution of fragments, one of the following methods should be used:

1. Continuous traction in a Thomas splint or knee flexion splint (Figs. 66 and 67 a). If this is done the best method is by Steinman pin through the os calcis or lower tibia. Skin traction should not be used in fractures below the knee. It is quite painful, is rarely effective and may cause skin eruption from irritation by the adhesive plaster which will prevent or delay open operation if traction should prove unsuccessful.

2. Two pins may be inserted well above and below the break (Fig. 67 b) and the upper pin fastened to the sides of a Thomas or similar splint

by means of pin lugs (Fig. 58 b). Traction is then applied to the lower pin until the fragments are pulled and manipulated into position when the lower pin is fastened to the sides of the splint by pin lugs. If the posi-

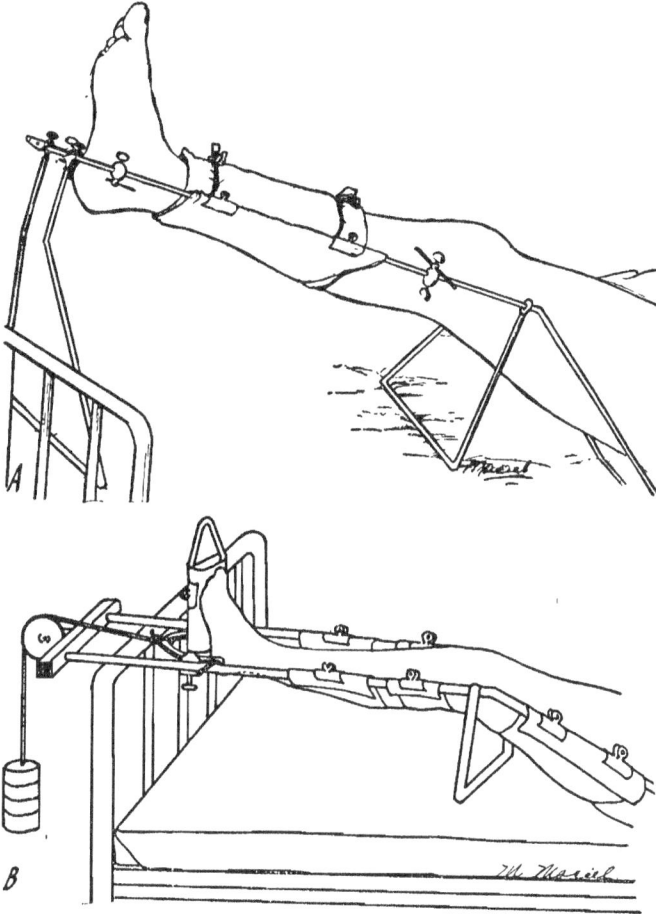

FIG. 67 a) Knee flexion splint used for fixation. Two or more pins are inserted through the tibia alone or through the tibia and os calcis and are locked to the sides of the splint with pin lugs. b) Knee flexion splint for traction. Traction by means of a pin through the os calcis. Skin traction for fractures below the knee is never effective.

tion is satisfactory, and when swelling has subsided, the leg may be incased in plaster, the pins being incorporated in the cast and cut off even with the plaster, when the latter has hardened.

3. Open fixation with plate, band, bone peg, or wire.

SPIRAL OR TORSION FRACTURE OF THE
TIBIA AND FIBULA (FIG. 68)

This particular fracture is fairly common and is produced by torsion of the leg as follows: When the foot is firmly fixed on the ground and the body twists suddenly, the tibia is twisted in two somewhere in its lower third and the form of the break is a long spiral or oblique fracture surface. This throws the entire body weight on the fibula which is broken by the weight and tortion in its smallest and weakest part, which is just below the head of the bone.

SYMPTOMS

Point tenderness, crepitus and mobility may be elicited in the tibial fracture, but the mobility will be slight for the reason that the fibula is broken at a distance from the fracture in the tibia. The fibular fracture may be suspected from the point of tenderness at the upper end. The radiogram which shows the fracture of the tibia may often fail to disclose the break in the tibia unless the film includes the knee joint. Its presence may be suspected, however, when the fracture of the tibia shows some shortening and no break in the fibula is shown.

TREATMENT

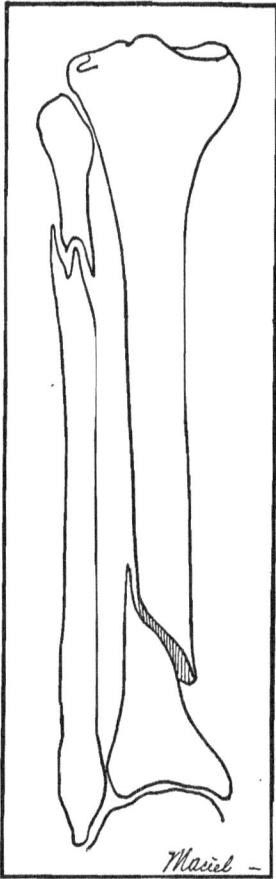

FIG. 68. Spiral or torsion fracture of the tibia and fibula.

This fracture is rarely reducible, for the reason that the broken fragments of the fibula are almost invariably firmly engaged by the pressure in their long axis. When the fragments of the fractured tibia are in good apposition with little overlapping, the entire leg may be incased in a cast just as it is. Care must be taken, however, to have this cast go well above the slightly flexed knee and that the foot is not rotated off its proper axis.

When the position of fragments is not good, and the leg is shortened somewhat, open fixation should be done without delay. Attempts at reduction or improvement in position are almost invariably futile. *Prob-*

ably the best and firmest fixation can be made with a *Parham Martin band.* Another occasional method is to transfix both fragments after reduction with a pin or nail, which is permitted to protrude through skin and cast, from which position it can be removed in four to six weeks. These fractures should be immobilized eight weeks and weight should not be borne for twelve weeks.

Fractures of the tibia and fibula should have the knee immobilized for at least four weeks and complete fixation of the break should be maintained for eight weeks. As a rule, if union is firm *and the fracture is transverse or slightly oblique,* adult patients may start weight bearing in ten weeks. Children may start weight bearing two or three weeks earlier. *When the break is comminuted or oblique,* it is safer to delay weight bearing until twelve to fourteen weeks pass. A frequent site for delay of union is the lower third of the tibia and it is not uncommon for some mobility to persist much beyond the usual time in this situation. When this occurs, the leg should be supported in a light boot cast and *cautious weight bearing and stamping with the heel* for several weeks will often stimulate the growth of callus.

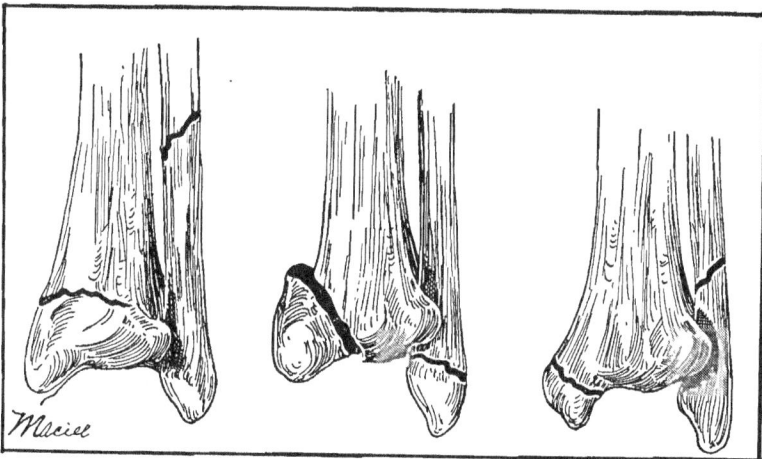

FIG. 69. Types of Pott's fracture.

POTT'S FRACTURE (FIG. 69)

Two common general types of injury take place in and about the ankle joint as a result of forcing the joint laterally beyond physiologic limits.

1. Inversion injury. The common inversion injury is the sprain of

the ankle in which the external lateral ligament is stretched or torn. Occasionally, the ligament holds and the external malleolus is fractured by avulsion.

2. The eversion accident. In this one of three things happened on the inner side of the ankle:

    a. The internal lateral ligament is stretched or torn.

    b. The inner malleolus is avulsed.

    c. The lower end of the tibia is fractured obliquely (Fig. 69).

Any one of these injuries permits the ankle to evert strongly and the astragalus, pressing against the inner side of the external malleolus, causes the fibula to break somewhere within the lower three inches of that bone.

This fracture was described by the British surgeon, Percival Pott in 1790 and in Anglo-Saxon countries is usually spoken of as the *Pott's fracture*. The French surgeon, Dupuytren, described the same condition in 1830 and in European continental countries the injury is usually called *Dupuytren's fracture*. While the two conditions described were not identical, both had reference to eversion types of fracture and both are clinically similar.

Occasionally, the direction of force is posterior as well as lateral and the posterior portion of the tibia is broken off obliquely and a triangular piece is broken off the posterior portion of the lower end of the fibula. The detachment of the two pieces of tibia and fibula permits the astragalus to dislocate posteriorly off the articular surface of the tibia. This type of fracture was described by F. J. Cotton of Boston in 1915 and is frequently referred to as the *Cotton fracture* or tri malleolar fracture.

SYMPTOMS

In Pott's fracture, the ankle joint appears widened. The foot is everted. Great swelling appears promptly. Point tenderness is felt over the internal malleolus and over the fibula just above the malleolus.

TREATMENT

Accurate and complete reduction is imperative if the foot is displaced laterally or posteriorly. When the axis of the foot and leg do not coincide, weight bearing causes strain on the foot and aggravation of the deformity and tendency to increase the angulation.

Local anesthesia is usually quite successful but *injections must be made on both sides* of the ankle into both fractures.

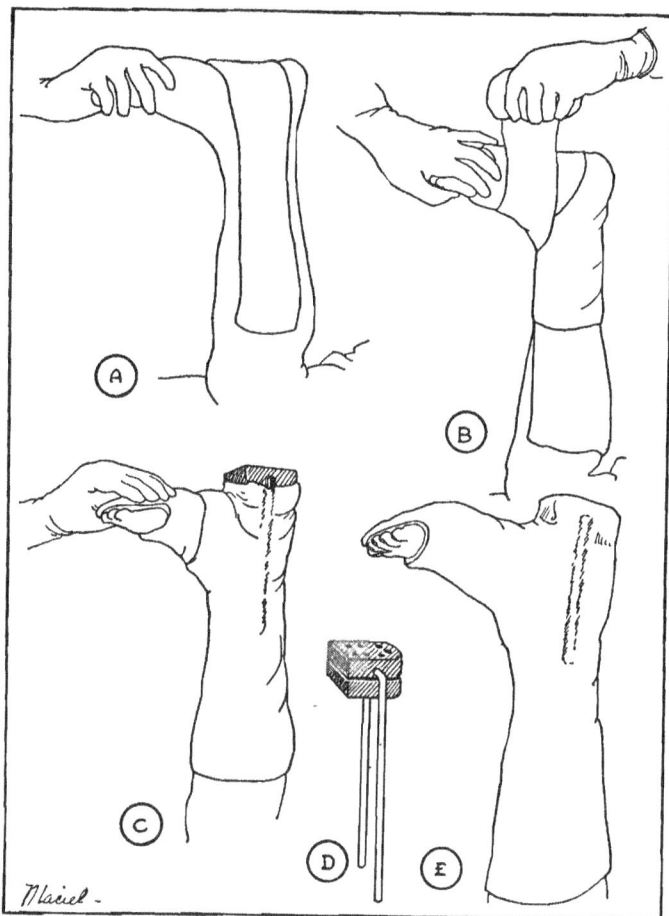

FIG. 70. Author's method of reducing a Pott's fracture. Applying cast with rubber heel. a) Patient face down on table. Knee is flexed to a right angle and fracture is reduced by internal rotation of foot and flexion of ankle. Reduction is easily maintained with one hand by an assistant and little interference with person applying plaster. A "sugar-tongs" splint is applied to the leg without any padding. b) The entire leg is covered with plaster. c) Two superimposed rubber heels held by a wire. d) are placed over the heel and the wires and sides of the heel are covered with plaster. e) Completed dressing.

REDUCTION

It is necessary to flex the knee to a right angle to relax calf muscles. The foot is then grasped about the instep, drawn forward, flexed to 90° and inverted, and the dressing is applied in this position. *All of this is best accomplished by turning the patient on his face and flexing the knee to a right angle* (Fig. 70). In this position, the knee rests on the table and the leg extends upward at 90° to the table and pressure downward on the foot makes counter pressure by the knee on the table. Reduction is very simple and easy in this position. It is readily maintained by an assistant who grasps the foot by the instep, inverts it and presses downward, flexing the foot to a right angle. This position is not fatiguing to the assistant and his hand does not interfere with the application of plaster.

By all odds the best splint is plaster. A molded plaster splint starts below the knee and covers both sides of the leg ("sugar tongs" splint), and a second splint covers the sole projecting beyond the toes and extends up over the posterior side of the leg. This constitutes the *Stimson dressing.* The splints should be bandaged into place and the leg should be sharply elevated. When swelling has begun to subside, the splints may be covered with a plaster bandage.

Böhler uses a dressing as described, but the plaster is unpadded. In a day or two an iron stirrup is fastened in the cast and on this the patient walks. Our practice is to fasten by means of plaster and a wire loop, a rubber heel on the heel of the cast and on this the patient bears weight. Either of these methods gets the patient about without crutches and reduces the period of convalescence.

Weight should not be borne on a Pott's or Cotton fracture sooner than six weeks (except in a walking cast). When the foot has not been sufficiently everted, it is often helpful and gives comfort if the inner side of the heel is elevated ⅛ to 3/16″.

SEPARATION OF THE LOWER EPIPHYSIS OF THE TIBIA

In children, usually before the 17th year, the lower epiphysis of the tibia may slip forward or backward as a result of injury. Reduction can usually be accomplished without difficulty and splinting is the same as a Pott's fracture.

DISLOCATION OF THE ANKLE

"This articulation which is formed by the tibia and fibula and astragalus with their cartilages and synovial membrane is so strongly protected by the form of the joint, and the numerous ligaments connecting these bones, that great violence is necessary to produce a dislocation, and when it does occur, it generally is accompanied by fracture, the ligaments offering more resistance than the bones." *Sir William Astley Cooper,* 1831.

Lateral dislocation without fracture is practically impossible. Anterior and posterior dislocations are rare injuries. The deformity is easily recognized if seen early. Reduction is accomplished without great difficulty under anesthesia. X-ray is necessary to exclude fracture.

FRACTURE OF THE ASTRAGALUS

This is a rare accident, usually associated with fracture of the os calcis. *It cannot be diagnosed except by x-ray.* Treatment is similar to fracture of the os calcis.

FRACTURE OF THE OS CALCIS

This injury nearly always results from falls on the heel. It is a fairly common industrial accident, seen in scaffold workers, such as painters, carpenters, steel erectors and tree surgeons. The injury is frequently bilateral.

SYMPTOMS

Great swelling comes on promptly. The heel appears widened. Point tenderness is elicited by pressing the heel between the thumb and forefinger and by pressing on the bottom of the heel. Ecchymosis appears early and is most evident below the malleoli. This injury is apt to cause considerable impairment in the form of constant pain on weight bearing, and hyperfatigability due to muscle strain and from endeavoring to favor the painful foot. Industrial commission statistics show that in 30 per cent of cases of this injury, some permanent partial disability persists.

Several varieties of calcaneal fractures are seen:

1. The bone may be broken across from above down.
2. Comminuted fractures with breaks in several directions.
3. Crushes in which the bone is flattened and widened.

Normally a line touching the upper border of the calcaneo-astragalus articulation intersects a line touching the uppermost prominences of that portion of the heel behind the calcaneo-astragalus joint at an angle of about 30°. In fractures of the os calcis, this angle will be greatly diminished so that, in some cases, the two lines coincide. By this, the normal arch of the foot is diminished or obliterated and the muscular balance of the foot is impaired (Fig. 71).

TREATMENT

No treatment need be applied early other than high elevation of the foot, and sedatives for the reason that extreme swelling and ecchymosis is almost immediate and a dressing will almost certainly soon become uncomfortably tight and fracture blebs are common. When swelling has about subsided, reduction and fixation should be attempted.

While accurate replacement of comminuted fragments is rarely possible, the arrangement of the displaced pieces can often be improved so as to correct *first,* the spreading of the heel; *second,* the flattening of arch.

The lateral spreading may be improved by gently malloting after

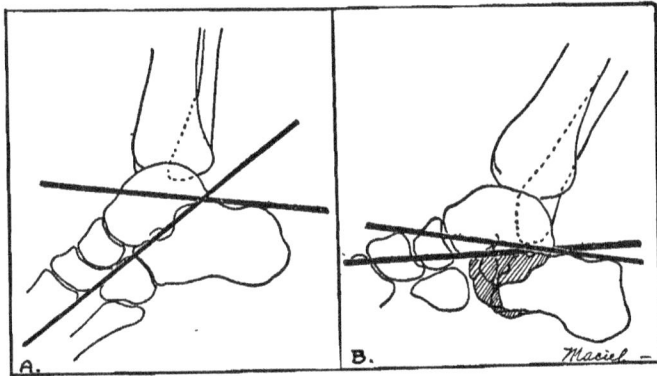

FIG. 71. Fracture of the os calcis. a) Lines show normal inclination of plane of articular surface of bone with plane of body of bone. b) Showing alteration of these planes when os calcis is fractured and depressed.

the manner of *Cotton.* The heel is laid on the outer side on a sand bag, a pad of felt is laid on the medial surface, and the fragments are malloted into position with a wooden mallot. *Probably a better method* is by clamping with a cabinet maker's C clamp or Böhler's redresseur. The flattening of the arch and restoration of the calcaneo-astragaloid angle is done by first inserting a pin through a firm portion of the os calcis, as far back as possible. With the knee flexed and firmly held in some sling or frame, traction is made downward and backward and an unpadded cast is applied incorporating the pin. Weight bearing should not be permitted . in less than three months. A special shoe with arch support is often necessary for comfort. Disability is due to:

1. Derangement of muscle balance in the sole of the foot, traumatic flat foot.
2. Traumatic arthritis of the astragalo-calcaneal joint.

3. Impingement on the peroneous longus tendon by a laterally displaced fragment.

Modified shoes, exercise, and suitable employment will often improve the first class. A subastragaloid arthrodesis is often necessary to relieve the constant discomfort in the second class. Operative removal of the offending fragment frequently gives prompt relief in the third class. This procedure was explained and advocated by *Magnuson*. In many cases, however, particularly bilateral fractures, pain, disability and general undermining of morale persist to a degree out of all proportion to the original injury.

FRACTURES OF THE TARSAL BONES

These occur from falling weights, run over accidents and wrenches where one part of the foot is held and force is applied to the free portion. The bones most frequently involved are the navicular and cuboid. Both of these bones are subjected to varieties of fractures and dislocations.

Swelling is extreme and early so that no accurate diagnosis can be made except by x-ray. Reduction may be made by clamping, molding and manipulation, and should be maintained with a cast from toes to the knee. Occasionally, a pin inserted in the heel may be used for traction and then imbedded in the cast to maintain position. Comminuted fractures and dislocations of the tarsus are often difficult or impossible to replace accurately. *There are few fracture problems in which experienced judgment and good understanding of the mechanics and anatomy involved are so important.* A working man with a constantly painful foot is very seriously impaired.

FRACTURE OF THE METATARSALS AND PHALANGES

These fractures are often difficult to detect because of the prompt swelling. Stimson's sign is usually a valuable one when the more definite symptoms are absent. A plaster boot is the best dressing, though when displacement is not great, mere abstinence from weight bearing is all that is required until pain has subsided.

When reduction is not possible, or the fracture is oblique, a Banjo splint imbedded in a plaster boot is *an excellent apparatus*. Traction may be made by rubber bands attached to wires or nails through the toes.

REFERENCES

BÖHLER, LORENZ: Treatment of Fractures. Baltimore, William Wood & Co., 1936.

CALDWELL, JOHN A. Spiral Fracture of the Tibia and Fibula. *Ann. Surg.*, 75: 717, June 1922.

CALDWELL, JOHN A.: Treatment of Fractures in the Cincinnati General Hospital. *Ann. Surg.*, 97: 170, *et seq.* Feb. 1933.

CONWELL, H. E.: Acute Fracture—Dislocations About the Ankle Joint. *Ann. Surg.*, 89: 439, March 1929.

CUBBINS, W. R. CONLEY, A. H. and SEIFFERT, G. S.: Fractures of Lateral Tuberosities of Tibia, etc. *Surg., Gynec. & Obst.*, 48: 106, Jan. 1929.

DUPUYTREN, G.: *Clinical Lectures on Surgery.* Trans. by A. D. Doane. Philadelphia, De Silver & Thomas, 1833.

GRISWOLD, R. A.: Major Fractures of the Tibia and Fibula. *Surg., Gynec. & Obst.* 58: 900, May 1934.

POTT, PERCIVALL: *Chirurgical Works.* London, J. Johnson, 1790. 3 Vol.

SPEED, KELLOGG: A Discussion of Pott's Fracture with Complications Based on a Series of 208 Cases. *Surg., Gynec. & Obst.*, 19: 73, July 1914.

Chapter XI

FRACTURES AND DISLOCATIONS OF THE SPINE

FRACTURES of the vertebrae require different judgment and treatment, *depending on whether or not the cord is damaged. When the cord has escaped,* the problem consists in restoring the alignment insofar as this is possible, and maintaining fixation until healing can take place. Failure to secure and maintain fixation for sufficient time often results in prolonged or permanent pain from muscle spasm or nerve root pressure or, occasionally, cord pressure from late shifting or compression of fragments.

When the cord is not affected: Cervical Region: These are brought about by falls on the head, diving accidents, twists, and jerks of the neck. In many cases the injury is not immediately disabling and the patient seeks advice for persistent pain and restricted motion. In x-ray diagnosis of these injuries, antero-posterior films often fail to show any abnormality, since the displacement is usually forward or backward, but lateral views disclose it promptly.

The common lesion is angulation of one vertebra on another, with partial crushing of the body and fracture of one or both laminae and dissengagement of one or both articular processes. Severe pain and sensory disturbances in one of both arms may be felt as a result of root compression.

TREATMENT

This should be instituted as soon as possible. Reduction is often possible by manipulation. This should only be done by one thoroughly familiar with the proper manoeuvers since uncautious or wrongly planned movements may result in cord injury. The proper successive steps for reduction have been well described by Langworthy, Taylor and others and consist in traction, hyperextension, lateral flexion and rotation. Deep general anesthesia is necessary and the movements should be checked at once by x-ray before the patient has reacted from anesthesia since reduction is often unsuccessful and must be repeated.

After reduction, some form of traction must be applied. Various forms of bridles and loops have been in use to make traction on the head, but all are extremely uncomfortable, are apt to cause pressure sores on occiput or chin, and are comparatively ineffective. In the past few years skeletal traction by means of several types of tongs or wire loops threaded through adjacent holes in the skull have come into use and their employment enables one to keep up effective traction for weeks. After traction for six weeks, the neck should be immobilized by a plaster cast covering head, neck and shoulders, or a Thomas collar. Some form of fixation should be continued for three months.

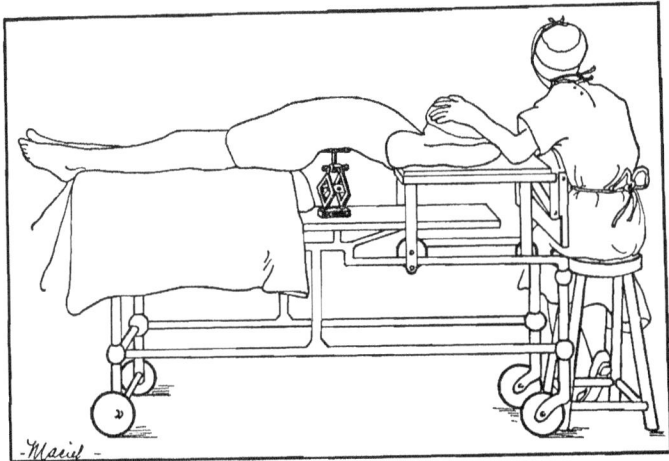

FIG. 72. Automobile jack method of hyperextension of the spine. Patient rests on Hawley table and a box or he may have his shoulder on one table, his buttocks on another and the jack on a stool between them. Adapted from Ryerson, E. W. Automobile Hyperextension of the Spine. *J.A.M.A.* 103, 562, Aug. 23, 1934.

Fractures and dislocations of *the thoracic and lumbar spine* are best treated as follows: Under general anesthesia, firm traction is made by four persons, one at each shoulder and one on each leg. At the same time the spine is strongly hyperextended. A good method is as follows: The patient is placed on two tables separated sufficiently to just admit the shoulders to rest on one and the buttocks on the other. In this position he is stretched and the back hyperextended. This may be done by laying the patient's face down when the hyperextension is accomplished by gravity, or he may be placed face upwards and hyperextended by a sling about the body, fastened overhead, or by a support pressing on the injured vertebra. An automobile jack is excellent for this purpose (Fig. 72). A cast is then applied from shoulders to buttocks with the spine strongly hyperextended. This is worn for three months and should be followed by a brace for six months.

Failure to treat compression fractures of the vertebral bodies or inadequate treatment is apt to be followed by permanent restriction of movement and pain in the back. This is a common cause of impairment after industrial accident. When pain persists to such a degree as to be incapacitating, a fusion operation should be considered. While this will be followed by some rigidity of the spine, existence may be made tolerable.

FRACTURES AND DISLOCATIONS OF THE SPINE
WITH CORD DAMAGE

Complete destruction of the cord is followed by: (1) complete motor and sensory paralysis below the lesion; (2) absence of all reflexes; (3) rapid development of bed sores; (4) complete paralysis of bladder and rectal sphincters.

When the cord injury is in the cervical region, a single or bilateral *Horner's syndrome* may be observed (contraction of the pupil with narrowing of the palpebral fissure). If the lesion is not high enough to paralyze the arms (below the third cervical vertebra), the arms may be partially paralyzed and have painful areas from root symptoms. Respiration is entirely diaphragmatic because of paralysis of the intercostal muscles.

Incomplete lesions of the spinal cord: These show variable symptoms, depending on the nature of the injury and its location. The causes of an incomplete lesion may be direct localized damage from penetration by a bone fragment or contusions of the cord followed by hemorrhage into the cord substance and edema.

Localized cord injury on one side is often followed by the Brown-Sequard syndrome. In this there is seen homolateral weakness with increased reflexes and spasticity and contralateral loss of pain and temperature sense.

Hemorrhage into the cord or hematomyelia has as *its most striking symptom: dissociation of sensation.* The pain and temperature fibres which decussate in the central portion of the cord are injured and consequently these sensations are lost or impaired. The fibres carrying the sense of touch ascend in the posterior columns and are often spared so that the patient retains the sense of touch but does not recognize pain and temperature. With these symptoms is muscular impairment with spasticity due to interference with the pyramidal tracts.

Concussion of the cord or impact lesions sometimes follow gunshot wounds which strike the spine but do not damage the cord directly. However, the cord is seriously damaged by the hydrostatic commotion and jar so that there is complete local disintegration. The symptoms are those of complete cord severance.

TREATMENT OF THE CORD INJURIES

A patient who has received a cord injury should have a thorough and detailed neurologic examination *at the earliest possible moment* and this should be recorded in order that changes indicating progress of the lesion may be noted. The procedure is as follows:

1. The patient should be completely stripped.
2. Breathing should be observed to note if the intercostal muscles are active.
3. Examine the spine for deformity, point tenderness, swelling, and hematoma.
4. Examine muscular action in the arms and legs.
5. Examine sensations, pain with a pin point, touch with a tuft of cotton, temperature with hot and cold test tubes.
6. Rectal examinations should be made to determine if sphincteral tone remains.
7. Deep and superficial reflexes should be examined.
8. Lateral and antero-posterior x-rays should be made.

When early examination indicates *a complete lesion,* no immediate radical treatment should be attempted. Patients with severe spinal lesions are easily thrown into severe or fatal shock if rough manipulations or operation are performed. A cord suffering complete severance or transverse damage never regenerates and recovery is hopeless. When this lesion is in the cervical region, a fatal outcome can be certainly predicted. A fairly accurate rule is one which says that a patient lives one day for every cervical vertebra broken and injuring the cord, e.g., death will occur on the fifth day if the lesion is at the level of the fifth cervical vertebra. Death is due to respiratory paralysis which results from ascending edema reaching the phrenic center in the cord and causing paralysis of the diaphragm. Death is preceded by *a sharp rise in temperature,* as high as 112°, which is due to involvement of the thermal regulating centre in the medulla. This is spoken of as the preagonal rise and *can be considered a sure sign of impending dissolution.*

When the lesion is lower, in the thoracic or lumbar region, while hope for recovery of function is hopeless, death may be delayed by good nursing. The principal difficulties come from bed sores and bladder infection. Development of bed sores should be combated by frequent turning, massage and rubbing of the skin, and the use of air cushions and mattresses. Cystitis and ascending urinary infections of the kidneys are best prevented by tidal bladder distension described by Monro. Repeated catheterization will inevitably be followed by cystitis and will require frequent bladder irrigations and a continuous catheter or cystotomy for its treatment. Death is due to sepsis from bed sores or bladder or renal infection or some intercurrent infection due to prolonged invalidism.

Incomplete lesions will often puzzle the most experienced to decide appropriate treatment. When the x-ray shows the cord pressed upon by a displaced vertebra, manipulation should follow with the hope that the dislocated segment may be reduced. When this is not possible, a laminectomy should be made to relieve pressure on the cord. Depressed laminae should be elevated by open operation.

It is not possible to tell how much damage is due to direct trauma and how much to secondary edema and hemorrhage. Doubt in these cases should be resolved in favor of conservatism. Surprising recoveries have followed cord injuries which on first examination seemed almost complete. A useful observation can be made by spinal puncture. When the puncture shows a spinal block, when the Queckenstedt test is positive, the lesion should be explored.

REFERENCES

BROOKES, T. P.: Dislocations of the Cervical Spine. *Surg., Gynec. & Obst.* 57: 772, Dec. 1933.

CRUTCHFIELD, W. G.: Further Observations on Treatment of Fracture. Dislocations of the Cervical Spine with Skeletal Traction. *Surg., Gynec. & Obst.,* 63: 513-517, Oct. 1936.

DAVIS, A. G.: Manipulative Reduction in Fractures of Spine. *Am. J. Surg.,* 15: 325, 1932.

DUNLOP, JOHN: Connection of Compressed and Impacted Fractures of the Vertebrae. *J. Bone & Joint Surg.*, 15: 153, Jan. 1933.

LANGWORTHY, M.: Cervical Vertebra Dislocations. *J. A. M. A.*, 94: 86-89, Jan. 1930.

MUNRO, DONALD. The treatment of the urinary bladder in cases with injury of the spinal cord., *Am. J. Surg.*, 1937, 38: 120-136.

MUNRO, DONALD, and HAHN, J.: Tidal drainage of the urinary bladder. *New England J. Med.*, 212: 229-239, 1935.

RYERSON, E. W.: Automobile Jack. Hyperextension of Spine. *J. A. M. A.*, 103: 562, Aug. 25, 1934.

Chapter XII

FRACTURES OF THE SKULL
AND HEAD INJURIES

FRACTURES of the skull in themselves are of little importance. The problem which concerns the surgeon is the location and kind of damage which the brain has sustained. The skull fracture, if one is present, gives valuable information as to the degree and direction of the injuring force.

Brain injury from trauma to the head occurs in five ways: (1) bruising or laceration of the cortex; (2) hemorrhage within or outside the dura; (3) disarrangement of the normal circulation of the blood and cerebrospinal fluid; (4) elevation of intracranial pressure by bleeding within the skull and edema of the brain; (5) jarring and commotion in the cortical cells, called concussion.

The brain is encased in the skull which is inelastic, hence anything which causes the brain to swell or causes hemorrhage within the head makes pressure on the brain. The brain itself is not compressible and the ventricular system and subarachnoid spaces are constantly filled to capacity with cerebrospinal fluid, consequently the effect of increased intracranial pressure is to diminish the capacity of the blood vessels and so reduce the blood supply to the brain.

From these statements, it follows that symptoms of brain injury consist of: (1) Concussion; (2) local symptoms, i.e., those due to localized brain injury; (3) symptoms of intracranial pressure. To these must be added the associated external evidence of injury, such as scalp lacerations, ecchymosis of the eyelids, bleeding from one or both ears or nostrils, and hematoma of the scalp.

1. Concussion has not been satisfactory explained, but is believed to be due to changes in capillary circulation of the cortex and molecular cortical disorganization due to jarring. In its mildest form, concussion is not associated with loss of consciousness, but with dizziness, weakness, slow pulse, pallor, and sweating. These symptoms may be evanescent and leave no after effect other than headache. Severe injury may cause transient or prolonged coma, followed by a variable period of confusion and disorientation. A common sequel to a severe concussion is obliteration

of all memory of events causing or preceding the accident which brought about the condition.

2. Local symptoms. These are of two kinds, irritative and paralytic, and are shown in the parts controlled by the damaged cortical area. The irritative symptoms manifest themselves by muscular twitching, rigidity and localized convulsions. Paralytic symptoms are evidenced by weakness or paralysis in the part controlled by the damaged cortex. All focal symptoms are contralateral. Extensive incomplete injury or pressure on the side of a cerebral hemisphere will be followed by complete hemiparesis or hemiplegia which includes the facial muscles.

Damage to frontal lobes has indefinite symptomatology, but common typical ones are memory defects, alterations in conduct, disorders of the will and judgment. Lesions of the motor strip are shown by symptoms on the part of the arm and leg and, sometimes, the face. When the lesion is left-sided, various forms of aphasia are exhibited. Lesions of the parietal lobe often show the symptom of astereognosis. Complete lesions of one of the above types are apt to indicate severe cortical damage or considerable pressure by a clot or accumulation of cerebrospinal fluid. Weakness alone usually is associated with localized pressure of light degree.

The signs of intracranial pressure have been conveniently divided by Kocher into four degrees:

1. Slight elevation of pressure. This is shown principally by lethargy or slight stupor and little else.

2. Moderate intracranial pressure is shown by deep stupor though the patient can be aroused by painful stimuli. The pulse is slowed to as low as 50 or even 40 beats per minute. The blood pressure is elevated. Breathing becomes stertorous.

3. The state of compensation in which the patient is deeply comatose, cannot be aroused. Respirations assume the Cheyne-Stokes type, pulse is slow, but full and high pressure. If not relieved this is followed by:

4. State of decompensation in which the pulse is frequent and running, respirations are rapid and associated with moist rales in the chest, the surface is bathed in profuse perspiration, and the temperature is elevated sometimes to as high as 112°, the pre-agonal rise.

These signs can be interpreted as representing progressive medullary anemia. In the early stages the vasomotor, vagus, and heart centers respond to the stimulus of medullary anemia, but when the stage of decompensation has been reached, such response is no longer possible.

Associated symptoms. Ecchymosis of the eyes when not due to direct trauma, usually means fracture, forward at the base with bleeding into the orbit. Bleeding from the nose, when not due to fracture of the nasal bones, is apt to be associated with fracture through the cribriform plate of the ethmoid bone or into the frontal sinus. Occasionally, there will be a flow of cerebrospinal fluid. Bleeding from the ear or ears is associated with fracture of the temporal bone, and is *sometimes* followed by flow of cerebrospinal fluid. These fractures are *occasionally* followed by paralysis of the facial nerve of the peripheral type.

Ecchymosis over the mastoid process (*Battle's sign*) indicates fracture at the base into the temporal bone.

When first examined, when the effect of concussion is still present, often no reflex response can be obtained. Later the response is characteristic of upper motor neuron lesions, i.e., the abdominal and cremasteric reflexes are obliterated and pathologic reflexes such as Babinski, Chaddock and Oppenheim may be obtained. Pupillary reflexes as a rule are not impaired. A widely dilated pupil is usually indicative of severe pressure or cortical injury on the same side of the head as the dilated pupil.

The phenomenon known as conjugate deviation is sometimes seen. In this the head and eyes are turned toward the injured side of the brain. It is often associated with a dilated pupil in the eye on the injured side. Spinal puncture often gives valuable information about brain damage, the two most valuable signs being degree of bloodiness of the fluid and intracranal pressure. Bloodiness may be anything from a slight pinkish tinge to fluid which cannot be distinguished from pure blood by its color. Normal spinal fluid pressure is between 10 and 20 cm. measured by the water manometer or 9 and 16 mm. when measured by the mercurial manometer. Pressure above the last limits should be regarded as pathological. *When a spinal puncture is done, the pressure should always be measured with a manometer.* Estimation of pressure by the spurt or rate of flow is so inaccurate as to be valueless. While a spinal puncture may be helpful in arriving at a complete and accurate diagnosis and give useful date toward a prognosis, it should not be used as a routine measure to complete a record as is, for instance, blood pressure reading or pulse and respiration tabulation. Though comparatively free from danger, it often gives pain to a conscious patient and causes a semi-conscious patient to struggle. It should rarely be done on a patient in shock, an alcoholic patient or one who struggles excessively. In these conditions it may do harm and the pressure readings are not reliable indices of intracranial pressure when made under the above conditions.

INTRACRANIAL CONDITIONS BROUGHT ABOUT BY CRANIAL TRAUMA

1. Extradural hemorrhage. Hemorrhage between the dura and skull follows a localized blow which bends or fractures the skull sufficiently to tear a meningeal vessel, which continues to bleed and separate the dura from the skull until it compresses the brain at the point of injury and increases the intracranial pressure. The commonest sites of extradural hemorrhage are the temporal regions for the reason that in these areas the skull is thinnest and beneath these localities are the middle meningeal arteries and their branches. The original injury is often trivial, frequently not sufficient to fracture the skull.

SYMPTOMS

A short period of unconsciousness due to concussion usually follows the injury though this often does not occur. The patient soon recovers consciousness and often continues his work for a time, but in the course of a few hours, consciousness is again gradually lost. When examined in this state, he will be found to be hemiplegic on the side opposite the injury, the pupil is often dilated on the same side as the injury. If not already completely comatose, stupor is rapidly deepening. A spinal puncture will sometimes show only a faintly bloody fluid, but the fluid may be quite bloody from associated cortical injury and bleeding from the vessels in the cortex. The spinal pressure is always high, 30 to 50 cm. in the water manometer. Reflexes are exaggerated on the paralyzed side and pathologic reflexes are present. The slow pulse, high blood pressure, and stertorous respirations associated with high intracranial pressure are present. Unless the condition is promptly relieved, the outcome is rapidly fatal.

Intradural Hemorrhage. In this condition the blood accumulates within the dural sac, often between arachnoid and pia and mixes with cerebrospinal fluid. Often bleeding will follow trivial injuries, will stop spontaneously, but recur after weeks or months and assume serious proportions. When this latter series of phenomena occur, the cortex is covered with a partially organized clot which is frequently cystic at the centre. The condition has been given the names of chronic intradural hemorrhage and pachymeningitis hemorrhagica.

The symptoms are those of localized and general intracranial pressure. The opposite side is paralyzed or paretic, and other contralateral focal symptoms are present. Spinal fluid is quite bloody but pressure is not always high.

Intracranial Hygroma. Occasionally, cranial trauma causes a laceration of the arachnoid thus permitting escape of cerebrospinal fluid from the subarachnoid space into the subdural space. The escaped fluid accumulates until it makes sufficient pressure to cause symptoms. These symptoms are contralateral paresis and, if the pressure is left-sided, aphasia. The spinal fluid pressure may be normal or slightly elevated, and the fluid is often blood tinged. It is not, as a rule, grossly bloody unless there is associated cortical laceration.

Treatment of head injuries. When the injury is severe and especially when associated with shock, the principal indications are rest and prevention of radiation of body heat. It is better to use facilities present rather than to disturb the patient and allow dissipation of heat by long transportation, but, as soon as it can be done safely, he should be removed to some place where any emergency can be met. A restless patient may require a sedative, but if it can be avoided morphine or its derivatives should not be used, for the reason that they depress respiration and mask pupillary changes so that information from that source is worthless. One of the barbiturates hypodermically is probably the most useful drug. A scalp wound should be thoroughly cleansed, the hair about it should be shaved, and it should be débrided and closed under local anesthesia. Bleeding from the ear should be allowed to continue, not stopped by plugging the meatus. No irrigation should be used but the canal may be swabbed with an antiseptic on an applicator and a large sterile dressing placed over the ear to catch drainage.

Unless the patient is in severe shock, the head of the bed should be elevated 8 to 12 inches and the patient should be allowed a pillow. With the head raised, blood pressure in the cranial vessels is reduced. When consciousness is impaired or the patient is disoriented, he should be attended constantly. Pulse and respiration should be recorded every half hour, and blood pressure every two hours. When the pulse rate falls below 60 or rises above 120, the person in charge should be notified. Paralysis, weakness, muscular twitchings, *and any peculiar behaviour* should be recorded in detail. Spinal puncture should be done if the patient does not react in 12 hours, *or sooner if there is special indication for it.* A patient in shock should not receive a puncture because of the exposure necessary. Puncture of an intoxicated person or one very restless from his head injury may be injured by his resistance and the value of the information disclosed by the puncture is reduced. X-ray of the head should be deferred for the same reason. To obtain a good picture of the head, the patient must be either cooperative or comatose. When the nature and extent of the injury is not apparent by other examination, an x-ray film should be made as soon as possible. Complete films of the head should always include stereoscopic views with the injured side next the film.

When no focal signs appear, and consciousness does not return or the patient is disoriented or confused, a spinal puncture should be made. If the pressure is found to be high, enough fluid should be removed to reduce the pressure 50 per cent. The puncture should be repeated in 8 to 12 hours and this should be continued as long as the pressure remains elevated to any marked degree. Intracranial pressure is also reduced by giving 50 to 100 c.c. of 50 per cent solution of sucrose intravenously two or three times a day. Magnesium sulphate per rectum may be given daily for the same purpose, though its action is less prompt and effective. Glucose 50 per cent, 50 c.c., and sodium chloride 30 per cent, 100 c.c., may be given intravenously, but are less desirable than the sucrose.

Operative treatment. Compound depressed fractures should be thoroughly débrided and fragments should be elevated or removed *at the earliest possible moment.* Depressed fractures should be explored and the fragments elevated as soon as convenient. They do not require the immediate attention that is imperative in compound injuries. The following conditions call for exploratory craniotomy immediately: (1) Extradural hemorrhage; (2) intradural hemorrhage. The place of election for exploration is beneath the temporal muscle unless focal symptoms indicate another locality. If enlargement of the opening is necessary, it may be done by means of a cranial rongeur or by cutting an osteoplastic flap, if much room is needed.

As a rule, hygromas do not require immediate operation, *if the diagnosis can be definitely made.* However, any persistent focal symptoms call for exploration of the side involved as soon as uncertainty can be dispelled. Persistent high intracranial pressure should be subjected to exploration and, when closing the wound, a skull defect should be left beneath the temporal muscle to permit decompression.

Any patient with a head injury who shows a bloody spinal fluid or who is unconscious for any considerable period, or who bleeds from nose or ear, should be kept in bed under observation for at least ten days.

REFERENCES

BEEKMAN, FENWICK: Head Injuries in Children. *Ann. Surg.*, 87: 355, March 1928.

CUSHING and PUTNAM: Chronic Subdural Hematoma. *Arch. Surg.*, 11: 329-393, Sept. 1925.

GARDNER, WM. J.: Traumatic Subdural Hematoma. *Arch. Neurol. &* *Psychiat.*, 27: 847, April 1932.

KENNEDY, FOSTER and WORTIS, S. B.: How to Treat Head Injuries. *J. A. M. A.*, 98: 1352, April 16, 1932.

MASSERMAN, J. H.: Effects of Intravenous Administration of Hypertonic Solution of Dextrose. *J. A. M. A.*, 102: 2084, June 23, 1934.

MUNRO, DONALD: Diagnosis—Treatment and Immediate Prognosis of Cerebral Trauma. *New England J. Med.*, 210: 287, 1934.

NAFFZIGER, H. C.: Depressed Fracture of the Skull. *Surg., Gynec. & Obst.* 56: 476, Feb. 5, 1933.

NAFFZIGER, H. C.: Subdural Accumulation of Fluid Following Head Injury. *J. A. M. A.*, 82: 1751-1752, May 31, 1924.

TROTTER, WILFRED: Pacchymeningitis Interna Hemorrhagica. *Brit. J. Surg.*, 2: 271, 1914-15.

WEED, L. H. and McKIBBEN, P. S.: Pressure Changes in Cerebro Spinal Fluid—Following Intravenous Injections of Solutions of Various Concentrations. *Am. J. Physiol.*, 48: 512, May 1919.

Chapter XIII

DELAYED UNION AND FAILURE OF UNION OF FRACTURES

WHEN for any reason (other than a pathologic condition at the site of fracture) union has failed to become firm after the lapse of the usual period and x-ray fails to show deposit of callus, measures should be instituted to stimulate growth of callus. Obviously any possible cause should receive appropriate treatment, even though its bearing on the cause of the failure of union is not apparent. For example, rickets, diabetes, syphilis, tuberculosis, should receive appropriate systemic treatment for those conditions. Arteriosclerosis should be treated by proper measures to improve the circulation of the part. Among those most useful are posture, heat, massage and, when available, passive vascular exercise.

In our experience, little has been accomplished by diet and medication designed to increase the calcium and phosphorous metabolism. Among those tried have been calcium and phosphorous salts, cod liver oil, viosterol, haliver oil, and a high vitamin diet. Of course, deficient or incorrectly balanced nutrition should be corrected to improve general health, but little should be expected in the way of direct effect on callus deposit. Nor have we seen any consistent or striking effect following the use of any endocrine product.

Bone, like any other tissue, grows strong by use. After a fracture, bone function must be discontinued or diminished for a time in order to prevent movement of fragments, x-ray films taken after a several weeks' period of immobilization show the density of the bone reduced because of decalcification. To correct this and restore blood and lymph circulation, *function should be resumed as soon as consistent with stability*.

Massage and passive motion have a distinct use in preserving muscle tone and maintaining blood and lymph circulation. However, both of these measures must be used with care and judgment. *A good working rule is that which says passive motion that causes pain is harmful*. This rule is especially applicable when fracture is into a joint. In these cases rough or forceful motion breaks up adhesions, causes fresh bleeding and is apt to cause deposit of excessive callus which may obstruct joint motion after the fracture has united. The principal function of bone is to support stress, and when this cannot be done in physiologic manner, some substitute may be used which will stimulate callus. Percussion over the site of the fracture is often effective for this. A stick one foot long is thrust into a ball of yarn 2½ to 3 inches in diameter and with this used as a mallet, the patient is instructed to tap the fracture lightly several times daily until the area begins to feel uncomfortable or is slightly reddened. *When the bone is deep seated*, percussion is not feasible or effective, and in these cases slight trauma to the end of the bone answers the same purpose. *When a humerus is involved*, the elbow may be struck with the opposite hand in such a manner that the fragments are jarred together slightly. *In the case of a femur or tibia*, the patient may stand on the good leg and stamp the heel of the injured leg as many times as he can without causing great pain, and repeat several times a day. Also, when using crutches he should touch the foot of the injured leg without bearing full weight.

When, after these measures, x-ray still shows callus to be deficient or absent, *open procedure must be employed*. The most conservative of these is multiple drilling. The fracture is exposed and as many drill holes as possible are made through the ends of the bones. Insofar as possible the holes should be bored in an oblique direction so that each hole will pass through both fragments. The purpose of this is to form tunnels through which granulation tissue can grow and vascularize the eburnated avascular ends.

When this plan fails, *the last resort is a generous bone graft*, cut preferably from the opposite leg. The best form of this is as large an inlay graft as can be used, firmly fixed in place by bone screws. Intramedullary grafts interfere with the development of medullary callus and should not be employed for non-union.

It is rare that bones fail to unite after the methods described have been employed, but sometimes all measures fail. In these cases the patient must reconcile himself to the condition, wear a brace, or submit to amputation and apply a prosthetic appliance.

REFERENCES

BANCROFT, F. W.: The Use of Small Bone Transplants in Bridging a Bone Defect. *Ann. Surg.*, 67: 457, April 1918.

BRAINARD, DANIEL: Report of Thirteen Cases of Ununited Fractures Treated by Subcutaneous Perforation of the Bone. *Chicago Med. J.*, 50: 421, 1858.

CAMPBELL, W. C.: Ununited Fractures. *Arch. Surg.*, 24: 990, June 1932.

COTTON, F. J.: Technic in Use of Grafts in Cases of Non Union. *J. Bone & Joint Surg.*, 10: 94, Jan. 1928.

PREWITT, P. V. and EASTON, E. R.: Rationale of Bone Drilling in Delayed and Ununited Fractures. *Ann. Surg.*, 107: 303, Feb. 1938.

SPEED, KELLOGG: Non Union After Fracture. *Ann. Surg.*, 90: 574, Oct. 1929.

WATSON-JONES: Fractures and Other Bone & Joint Injuries. Baltimore, Williams & Wilkins, 1941, Page 26 et seq.

Chapter XIV

OPERATIVE TREATMENT OF FRACTURES

W HEN fractures of long bones cannot be reduced, fixation by open operation should be done as soon as the decision can be made. Such operation should only be done in a well organized operating room with complete facilities, by a surgeon thoroughly familiar with such operations, and who has the necessary instruments.

A bone operation requires the most rigid asepsis. When possible, the skin should receive sterilizing preparation *24 hours before* by thorough shaving, scrubbing, and application of a sterile dressing.

Before operation, an ample field should be cleansed and sterilized *again* and drapery should be applied in such a manner that it cannot be disarranged by manipulation of the part. Our custom is to roll two layers of previously autoclaved stockinet over the limb and through this the incision is made.

After making the skin incision, discard the knife, and clip towels to the wound margins with skin clips. In this way contact with the patient's skin by instruments or hands is prevented and no instrument is permitted in the wound which has touched skin. The incision should be ample in order to make forcible retraction or rough handling of tissue unnecessary. Hemostasis should be thorough throughout the operation. There should be as little hand contact with the wound as possible.

When the bone has been exposed and reduced, there are many methods of fixation. Which one will be employed *will depend upon the bone involved, the type of break, and the preference and experience of the operator.* The materials for fixation can be divided as:

1. Absorbable   a. Autogenous
                 b. Heterogenous
2. Non-absorbable   Plates, bands, wire and ivory or metal screws.

Autogenous material consists of pieces of bone taken from the patient and applied in a trough which bridges the fracture, or as an intramedullary dowel. Occasionally, strips of fascia are used for bone suture. Bone grafts require a special instrumentation: A motor saw is usually employed to cut grafts and their bed in cases of non-union or delayed union, the graft serving as a nidus for bone growth. The graft is anchored in place by means of metal or bone screws or ligatures of catgut or other absorbable material. Occasionally, bones are tied together by means of autogenous fascial bands which are threaded through holes drilled in the apposing ends of the bone.

Intramedullary dowels of autogenous bone are used most frequently in small bones, such as metacarpals or the radius and ulna for the reason that there is objection to the bulk of grafts applied to the surface. There is a theoretical objection to the use of any foreign body within the medullary canal because it displaces *the bone marrow,* an important substance necessary to bone growth and repair.

Heterogenous absorbable foreign material is usually catgut or kangaroo tendon used for lashing or suture of apposed bones. Beef bone or ivory may be used as intramedullary splints, as pegs or screws. Foreign bone inlays or applied bone plates are occasionally employed, but their bulk is an objection.

The foreign material used depends largely upon the nature of the break. Large deep seated bones, such as the humerus or femur, can be held by a metal plate of the *Lane or Sherman design,* fastened to the bone by means of screws. This is an adaptation of the mending plate used by cabinet makers. Smaller or superficial bones are often lashed together by tightly twisted wire. Many metals have been used, but stainless steel wire serves every purpose. Silver wire is not strong and is quite soft so that there is no particular reason for its selection. In the past few years research has demonstrated that metals which oxidise when buried in the tissues cause irritation and favor the development or persistence of infection. Also certain metals, combined as alloys, cause electrolytic reaction, which, often, is followed by an osteitis and consequent loosening of the fixation. Venable has demonstrated that any metallic fixation material should be electrolytically inert, and two different metals should not be used when fixing bones by internal splints.

When the fracture is very oblique a tight encircling band of steel, such as a Parham-Martin band, is excellent, is easy to apply and affords a firm fixation. Wire may be used the same way but wire does not afford as firm a fixation as the band. An encircling band of any sort should not be used on the bones of children where the bone has not attained full growth. As the bone grows it will surround the metal, which finally becomes imbedded in the bone and makes a weak place which is liable to fracture later.

No fixation applied to bone should be depended on for complete immobilization but the part should be immobilized with splints until union has taken place.

REFERENCES

The text books of Scudder, Key and Conwell, Speed, and Watson Jones all have excellent articles on *Open Treatment of Fractures*.

HENRY, A. K.: Complete Exposure of the Radius. *Brit. J. Surg.*, 1925, 13-506.

Also—Exposure of the Humerus and Femoral Shaft. *Brit. J. Surg.*, 1925, 12: 84.

SHERMAN, W. O. N.: Operative treatment of fractures. *J. A. M. A.*, 58, pp. 1557-1561, 1912.

VENABLE, C. S., STUCK, W. G., and BEACH, ASA: Effects on bone of the presence of metals; based upon electrolysis. Ann. Surg., 105, pp. 917-938, 1937.

Chapter XV

COMPLICATIONS AND SEQUELAE OF FRACTURES

THE commoner complications and sequelae to be anticipated are mentioned and discussed in connection with the particular fractures. However, after all fractures there are certain effects to be expected which are invariably present to a greater or lesser degree, and give rise to apprehension and impatience on the part of the patient and worry by the attending physician.

FRACTURE BLEBS

When a fracture is followed by considerable hematoma and swelling, large blebs or blisters are apt to form over the surface of the skin. The most frequent sites are about the elbow and ankle; situations where the soft tissue covering is shallow and the skin becomes tight very rapidly. They are not often seen over the thigh and upper arm, but are frequently found developed to great size over the elbow. The confining wall is extremely thin; it ruptures easily, thus allowing the viscid fluid to escape and soil dressings. The escaped fluid dries hard and, if not discovered, becomes infected with saprophytes and very foul. Later the skin may become infected and cellulitis follow.

The best deterrent of fracture blebs is early accurate reduction, after which the fractured member should be sharply elevated. If a cast or any confining dressing is applied, it should be loosened and as much of the member exposed as possible.

When blebs form, they should be evacuated, not by wide incision, *but by aspiration.* The outer wall of the bleb is the best covering of the weeping skin beneath and prevents dressings from sticking. If the blebs refill after draining, a good plan is to transfix carefully the blister with a sterile silk suture and leave the ends free; then any fluid which reaccumulates will drain off.

It is best not to apply dressings in contact with the blebs. The most satisfactory treatment has been to leave the part exposed and paint it with a 5 per cent solution of tannic acid in water, or gentian violet, 11 per cent.

The uninformed patient is prone to think that full function will be restored when all splints or apparatus are removed. He is surprised and alarmed when he finds motion of joints restricted, strength of muscles reduced, and that attempts to use the member cause it to become painful and swollen and tired with very little use.

The patient should be warned to expect these conditions and cautioned to restore function gradually. Energetic measures are certain to be followed by such great pain and disability that complete rest must be carried out until the part again becomes comfortable and a new start must be made.

Restricted motion follows practically invariably fixation of joints. When the fracture is remote from a joint, this is due to the prolonged rest of muscle with the invariably accompanying atrophy—and adhesions of adjacent sheaths of both muscles and tendons. Inactivity of muscle also causes stasis of lymph flow and loss of vascular tone which result in impairment of nutrition of all soft structures; and bone is affected to equal or greater extent. When the fracture is close to a joint, motion of the adjacent articulation may be further restricted by adhesions of tendons to sheaths, through compression by callus; by adhesions of synovial surfaces; and, occasionally, by deposit of callus into the joint.

All of these conditions may have their disappearance hastened by judicious physiotherapy in the forms of motion (active and passive) massage, and heat, cautiously applied and properly controlled.

Active motion, when possible, is always to be preferred to passive motion, for the reason that it is more gradual and stops short of producing pain.

Passive motion, *always,* should be used with care and gentleness by an experienced person and *should never cause pain.* A useful dictum popularized by John B. Murphy should never be forgotten—*"Passive motion which causes pain is harmful."* A painful session with an overenthusiastic operator is certain to be followed by so much soreness that no further efforts will be tolerated for several days and, when comfort has finally been restored, the movement will be found to be unimproved.

Passive motion under anesthesia is occasionally employed to break up adhesions. It is of the greatest value where the cause of restricted motion is not in, but about, the joint, and here it should be used only with caution, and by an operator with experience. It should never be employed when the cause of the restriction is organic (e.g., callus deposited in or near the joint, or bony ankylosis), nor should too great force be used to mobilize a fixed joint.

Heat is beneficial to improve blood and lymph supply and to reduce pain. A half hour application of heat before massage or passive motion makes the seance more comfortable and effective. It is best applied by infra-red rays, electric pad, hot water bottle or diathermy. The various electric methods are the most comfortable and effective. The seance should be fifteen to thirty minutes.

Swelling always follows removal of apparatus and resumption of function—probably on account of increased permeability of capillaries, due to lack of tone of all tissues. As would be expected, it is more evident in injuries affecting the lower extremities where the effect of diminished tonus is augmented by gravity. It is more extensive and persists longer in older than in younger persons and is, to some degree, proportional to the severity of injury and the period of immobilization. An adult, who has sustained a major fracture in a leg, may expect some edema of the member for at least six months. This will be increased by the upright position and use and will gradually diminish. It is almost invariably gone in the morning—to recur at night.

Massage is helpful to restore tone to muscles and thus give support to vessels. When the swelling is very uncomfortable, an elastic stocking or bandage gives comfort—or the application of a stocking of Unna's paste may give very effective support and does not interfere greatly with function.

Phlebitis occasionally follows fractures. It is more common during early convalescence but occasionally is seen late after movement has been begun. It is more frequently observed in the leg than in the arm—the saphena magna vein being most commonly affected.

The onset of phlebitis is first made known to the patient by severe sharp pain—usually in Scarpa's triangle or the popliteal space. Examination will show the leg as swollen, edematous, and tender to pressure along the course of the vein. When the affected vein is superficial, it may stand out and be palpable as a cord, and very painful to touch.

When phlebitis occurs—all motion, massage and manipulation should be stopped. The afflicted part should be oiled *gently*, elevated and immobilized, and wrapped in cotton or sheet wadding. This treatment should be continued until swelling subsides—until a collateral venous circulation has been established and the temperature has been normal for at least one week. By that time the clot will probably be sufficiently organized so as not to be dislodged and become an embolus.

Embolism, fat or blood clot, is *an occasional and most dreaded sequel of a fracture.* It may occur soon after the fracture or follow later manipulation. An embolus may cause sudden death by lodgement in a large cerebral, pulmonary, or cardiac vessel; or may cause lesser symptoms by infarction of the lung or cerebrum.

When infarction takes place the only treatment is absolute rest. Morphine should be given to insure this and to relieve pain and, if the infarct is pulmonary, the patient should be partially set up to relieve respiratory embarrassment.

Localized myositis ossificans or calcified hematoma occasionally occurs near a fracture. Its most common site is in the cubital fossa following fractures about the elbow joint, and the popliteal space. The calcified mass is seen by x-ray, and may often be felt and frequently blocks motion of the joint by its mechanical presence.

The mass may occasionally resorb to such extent that it no longer causes pressure or restricts motion. When this does not occur, removal should be considered.

Acute osteoporosis—also known as acute neurogenic bone atrophy and Sudeck's atrophy—was first described by Sudeck in 1902. Recently the importance and prevalence of this complication has been discussed and emphasized by Fontaine and Herrmann, and Frazier Gurd.

While this condition is seen most commonly following fractures about the wrist and ankle joints, it may follow lesser injuries in which no fracture occurs. It is not proportionate to severity of injury; being often observed when the fracture is so slightly displaced as to require no reduction.

In a normal course, immobilization is followed by subsidence of pain within two or three days. *When pain continues after this period, the possibility of acute osteoporosis beginning should be suspected.* The pain is apt to persist during the period of immobilization and after motion has been started. The pain is of a peculiar boring character and is most harassingly continuous. Like most pain associated with bone disorders, it is nearly always worse at night and frequently requires an anodyne to permit rest. On removal of the cast and, for weeks afterward, some swelling will be observed. This is usually not great. It does not pit on pressure and is often just enough to obliterate the grooves between the tendons. It is not generally associated with any marked change in color. *Careful palpation* will usually reveal slight elevation of temperature of the part, which will be confirmed by surface thermometer or thermocouple studies.

Roentgenographic study, which properly should consist of contrast plates made with the afflicted member and its fellow on the same plate with the same exposure, will reveal some degree of bone atrophy, sometimes as early as three weeks after injury. The appearance of the atrophy is characteristic. It differs from disuse atrophy in character, and appears much earlier. Where disuse atrophy is a uniform diminution of density, osteoporosis is a spotty or mottled irregularity of density which gives a mossy or "rotten wood" appearance to the part.

While acute osteoporosis is not common, it is sufficiently frequent to give rise to much misunderstanding. The common errors in diagnosis are disuse atrophy and neurosis, either of which cause a decided injustice to the patient—especially when compensation is a factor.

The cause of acute osteoporosis is not understood, and, consequently, its origin has given rise to much speculation. It is probably due to traumatic vasomotor nerve disturbance, a view which is given credence by the fact that the condition occasionally occurs in a hand or foot when the injury has been to some part of the limb higher up.

Since the etiology of acute osteoporosis is not understood, all treatment has been on an empirical basis, and none of this has been uniformly successful. Most patients affected develop some habit of motion or irritation of the affected member, such as finger drumming, slapping, foot tapping of the affected part, or some constant motion of the part. Any immobilization prevents this relief mechanism and makes the pain more intolerable. Usually any form of heat fails to relieve and often increases the pain.

Massage, passive motion, and as much active motion as the nature of the injury will permit is often helpful. When the pain persists and is intolerable, prompt subsidence has sometimes followed an arterial sympathectomy, though the explanation of how this brings about relief is not at all clear. This procedure has been used particularly by Leriche, Fontaine, and Herrmann and his associates. To be effective it must be employed early, before permanent changes have taken place in the bones and joint.

Occasionally, the condition goes on to extreme demineralization of the part with ankylosis of the joint.

REFERENCES

FONTAINE, R. and HERRMANN, L.: Post-traumatic Painful Osteoporosis. *Ann. Surg.*, 97: 26-63, February 1933.

FRASER, GURD: Sudeck's Atrophy. *Ann. Surg.*, vol. 99, March 1934.

LERICHE ET FONTAINE: Des Osteoporoses Doulereuses Post-traumatiques. *Presse méd.*, 1930, xxxviii, 617.

HERRMANN, L. and CALDWELL, JOHN A.: Diagnosis and Treatment of Post-traumatic Osteoporosis. *Am. J. Surg.*, Vol. 51, No. 3, March 1941.

MIDDLETON and BRUCE: Post-traumatic Dystrophy at Joints. *Edinburgh M. J.* 1934, xli, 49.

OPPENHEIMER: The Swollen Atrophic Hand. *Surg., Gyn. Obst.*, 1938, lxvii, 446.

SOUTAR SIMPSON: Post-traumatic Decalcification of the Foot. *J. Bone & Joint Surg.*, 1937, xix, 223.

SUDECK: Ueber die akute Entzundliche Knochenatrophie. *Arch. f. Klin. Chir.*, 1900, lxii, 147.

Chapter XVI

FIRST AID MEASURES AND EMERGENCY
TREATMENT OF FRACTURES

WHEN a patient who has met with an accident is first seen, *it is important not to make an examination or cause any movement which will cause pain or increase shock.*

Examination should be limited to that which is necessary to determine the presence or possibility of a fracture, and the patient should not be moved more than is necessary to get him to a place of safety or into shelter from exposure. Of Mr. Percival Pott, who described the *Pott's fracture,* and who showed keen practical surgical judgment and insight when he himself sustained a fracture of the leg in 1756, Sir James Earle, his son-in-law, successor, and biographer, gives the following account of the accident to Pott and his direction for his immediate treatment:

"As he was riding in Kent-street, Southwark, he was thrown from his horse, and suffered a compound fracture of the leg, the bone being forced through the integuments. Conscious of the dangers attendant on fractures of this nature, and thoroughly aware how much they may be increased by rough treatment, or improper position, he would not suffer himself to be moved until he had made the necessary dispositions. He sent to Westminster, then the nearest place, for two chairmen, to bring their poles; and patiently lay on the cold pavement, it being the middle of January, till they arrived. In this situation he purchased a door, to which he made them nail their poles. When all was ready he cause himself to be laid on it, and was carried through Southwark, over London-Bridge, to Watling-Street, near St. Paul's where he had lived for some time,— a tremendous distance in such a state! I cannot forbear remarking, that on such occasions a coach is too frequently employed, the jolting motion of which, with the unavoidable awkwardness of position, and difficulty of getting in and out, cause a great and often a fatal aggravation of the mischief."

When a person has sustained a fracture of a leg and the break is of such character that the slightest movement is painful, *he should not be*

moved until sufficient help is at hand to move him without severe pain,
and that should not be attempted until the conveyance to transport him
has arrived, and not then until sufficient splinting has been applied to
make it possible to lift and carry him without displacing fragments.

The army injunction to "splint 'em where they lie" has been responsible for saving many lives and relieving much pain. It is a good rule not
to move a patient from where he has fallen, unless it is necessary for
his safety or comfort, until his fracture can be splinted. When a patient

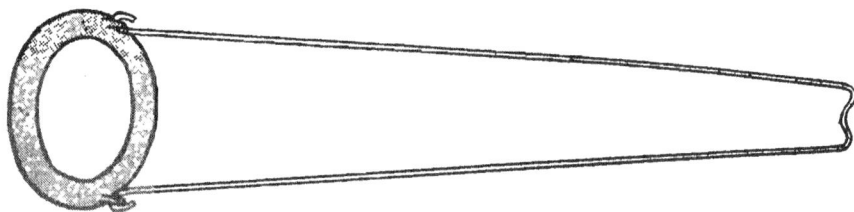

FIG. 73. Murray Jones' arm splint. From Kennedy, R. H. Transportation of the
wounded. *Bull. Am. Coll. Surg.* 17: 21, 1933.

has sustained a fracture at home, no good is accomplished, and much
harm may be done by helping the patient to walk or by carrying him
without any immobilization of his fracture and placing him to bed. It is
much better to leave him where he lies, make him comfortable with
pillows, cover him with blankets if he is chilly, and await the arrival of
the physician or person who understands handling the injured. A patient
can be examined and splinted just as thoroughly and effectively on the
floor as in bed and, after the true nature and extent of the injury have
been ascertained, he can be moved much more carefully and with
greater comfort.

One of the most serious fractures received about the home is that
near the neck of the femur. A frequent course of handling consists in
assisting the patient upstairs, with much suffering and shock, putting
him to bed, then calling a physician who often gets portable x-ray films.
If these show a fracture, the patient must be moved to a hospital where
good x-ray films can be taken and proper treatment instituted and carried out to completion. A more sensible and less harassing plan would
have been to *let the patient lie where he had fallen and not move him*
until means for transportation were at hand.

When it is necessary to carry a severely injured patient upstairs, if
there is nothing at hand which will serve as a litter (e.g., a narrow

door or a shutter) or if the stairs so turn that the use of a litter is impossible, the patient may be put in a stout chair and the rear bearer grasps the back of the chair near the top and the front bearer lifts by the front

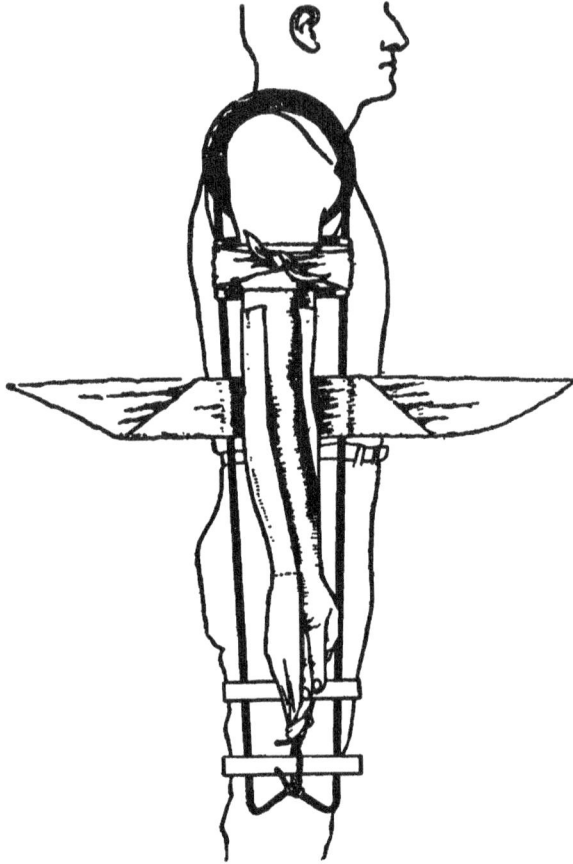

FIG. 74. Murray Jones' arm splint applied. U. S. Army method—traction is obtained by zinc oxide adhesive to the skin of the arm and forearm. The upper wooden silver prevents torsion of the adhesive on the hand, as traction is secured by twisting the rope. One triangular bandage only is applied, the second one is in position. The gauze bandage has not been applied over the adhesive. From *Red Cross Manual*.

legs and in this semi-reclining position, the patient can be carried upstairs by two strong persons in fair comfort.

When a patient must be transported, some means should be taken to prevent the pain and shock occasioned by the movement of the bones caused by the jolting and swaying of the vehicle. Pain associated with movement of a broken bone is due to the stretching and tearing of the periosteum. The best way to prevent this pain is by traction which tends to draw the two fragments apart. Splints of the Thomas type have proven their usefulness and effectiveness beyond question in both civil and military practice, and should be applied in fractures of the arm or leg. When the regular Thomas splint or some modification is not at hand, a traction splint may be improvised (Fig. 76). When material is at hand and the fracture can be located with sufficient accuracy, if 20

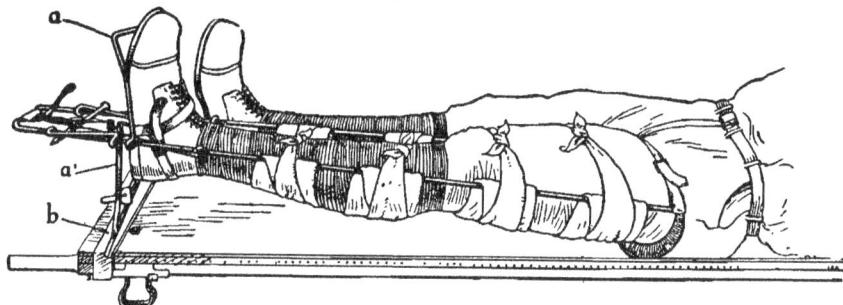

FIG. 75. Thomas splint applied. U. S. Army method—the ring of the hinged half-ring splint is made fast against the tuberosity of the ischium by tightening the anterior strap. Fixed traction is made by the adjustable traction strap or ankle hitch (Fig. 12). The extremity is secured to the side bars of the splint by four or more triangular bandages. The foot is supported by the foot rest (a). The splint support (a) is secured to the litter bar (b). The patient is now ready for transportation.

to 40 c.c. of 2 per cent procaine can be injected into the hematoma, the break will be rendered painless for about two hours and the patient can be transported in comfort. The author on two occasions has injected procaine into a fracture of the neck of the femur in senile females while they were lying on the floor in their homes, and then called an ambulance, moved them to a hospital, had x-ray films taken, reduced the fracture, and applied a cast before sensation had returned in the region of the fracture.

Fractures of the spine are always serious injuries. Ill-advised, hasty, or careless moving may easily shift fractured or displaced vertebrae sufficiently cause them to impinge on roots or the spinal cord if they have not already damaged those structures. When a person has met with an accident which has not rendered him unconscious but has prevented him from moving, a *spinal cord injury* should be suspected. Such a person should not be moved without a stretcher. A blanket should be slipped under him and *he should be cautiously dragged or slid by pulling on the blanket until he is pulled onto the stretcher.* If he must be moved a short distance without a stretcher, he should be carried face down on a blanket. Similar methods should be used and caution observed in fractures of the pelvis and serious abdominal injuries.

In all injuries proper measures should be used to combat shock. The best drug for this is *morphine,* which relieves pain and apprehension,

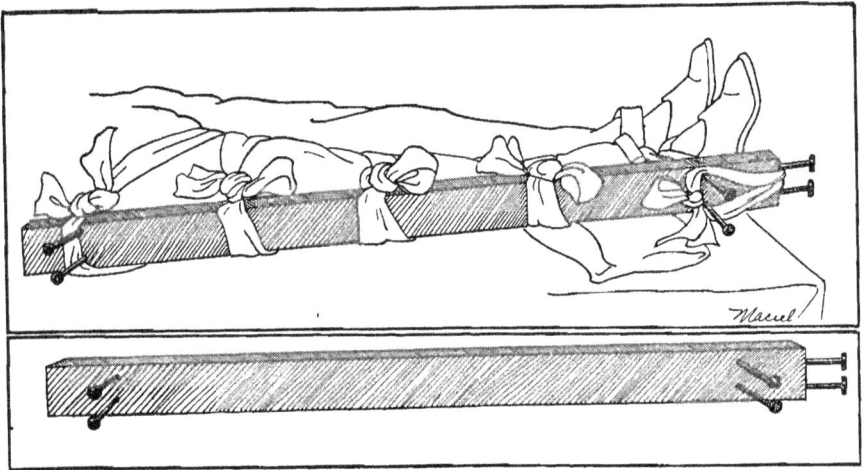

FIG. 76. Improvised transport splint for fracture of femur. A board 4″ x 4′ x ⅞″ has six nails driven in as illustrated. Such a splint reduces lateral motion and prevents the ends of the bone from rubbing together by traction. The effect is similar to that of a Thomas' splint.

slows the respiration, and diminishes shock. All methods which conserve heat and prevent its dissipation, diminish shock. When the transportation distance is to be considerable, blankets should be warmed before being thrown over the patient, hot water bottles placed about the legs and body, and lanterns under the litter may help considerably. As a rule, alcoholic beverages are best omitted. They cause the dilatation of peripheral vessels and so favor heat loss, and thus cause suspicion of alcoholism as a contributing factor.

When the *injury is to the head* and the patient is unconscious or stuporous, there should be as little movement as possible. *Neither morphine nor stimulants should be administered to a patient with a head injury.* Morphine may embarrass respiration already impaired by the brain injury or intracranial pressure. It causes contraction of the pupil so that observation of pupillary changes are worthless.

The head should be elevated somewhat so as to reduce intracranial hemorrhage. A scalp wound should have an aseptic dressing applied. *As soon as possible* the patient should be gotten to a place suitable for a complete and accurate examination.

REFERENCES

KENNEDY, R. H.: Emergency Treatment of Extremity Fractures. *New England J. Med.*, 207: 393-395, 1932.

FINDLAY, R. T.: First Aid for Fractures. *J. Bone & Joint Surg.*, 13: 701-708, 1931.

First Aid Text Book. American Red Cross. Philadelphia, P. Blakiston & Son Co., 1937.

KENNEDY, ROBERT H.: Transportation of the Injured. *Bull. Am. Coll. Surgeons*, 17: 21, 1933.

An Outline of the Treatment of Fractures. Chicago, American College of Surgeons, 1933.

YERGASON, R. M.: *Emergency Treatment of Fractures*. Hartford, Conn., Aetna Casualty Co.

APPENDIX

This table shows the time required for various stages of union and restoration of function.

The times given are only approximate and the figures are weeks.

BONE	FIRST APPEARANCE OF CALLUS	FIRM UNION	FULL FUNCTION
Phalanges, and metacarpals and metatarsals	2-3	3-6	6
Radius and ulna shaft	3	6-8	10-12
into elbow	3	5	12-14
into wrist	3	6	7-10
Humerus			
lower end	2-4	6	8
shaft	2-4	6	8
upper end	2-4	6	8-12
Pelvis	4	8	Weight bearing 8-16 wks.
Femur			
neck	12	24	60
intertrochanteric	4	12	16
shaft	6	12	14
supracondylar	6	12	14
Patella	6	6	6-12
Tibia and Fibula			
into knee	6	6	14
shaft	4	6	12
into ankle	6	6	12
Calcaneus	6	6	12-24

INDEX

This Book

A Manual of

THE TREATMENT OF
FRACTURES

By JOHN A. CALDWELL, M.D.

was set, printed and bound by The Collegiate Press of Menasha, Wisconsin. The type face is Linotype Caslon Old Face, set 11½ point on 13 point. The type page is 27 x 44 picas. The text paper is 70-lb. White Stonewall Eggshell. The binding is Du Pont, PXB-6, Color 7060 Linen, Grain satin-1, Finish Embossed. The jacket is Strathmore, Emissary Text, Apple Green, Antique Finish.

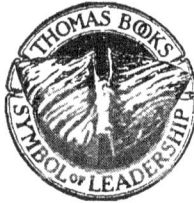

With THOMAS BOOKS careful attention is given to all details of manufacturing and design. It is the publisher's desire to present books that are satisfactory as to their physical qualities and artistic possibilities and appropriate for their particular use. THOMAS BOOKS will be true to those laws of quality that assure a good name and good will.

CPSIA information can be obtained
at www.ICGtesting.com
Printed in the USA
BVOW09s1439241017

498539BV00010B/115/P